1550

D1561819

Horizons in
Perinatal Research
IMPLICATIONS FOR CLINICAL CARE

CLINICAL PEDIATRICS, MATERNAL AND CHILD HEALTH

Series Editor: NORMAN KRETCHMER, Department of Pediatrics,
Stanford Medical Center, Stanford, California

Control of the Onset of Puberty, Melvin M. Grumbach, Gilman D.
Grave, and Florence E. Mayer

Horizons in Perinatal Research: Implications for Clinical Care, Norman
Kretchmer and Eileen Hasselmeyer

Horizons in
Perinatal Research

IMPLICATIONS FOR CLINICAL CARE

A Symposium Sponsored by the
Perinatal Biology and Infant Mortality Branch
National Institute of Child Health
and Human Development
Stanford, California

Norman Kretchmer, M.D., Ph.D.
and
Eileen G. Hasselmeyer, Ph.D., R.N.
scientific editors

A Wiley Biomedical-Health Publication

JOHN WILEY & SONS

New York   London   Sydney   Toronto

Library of Congress Cataloging in Publication Data

Main entry under title:

Horizons in perinatal research.

(A Wiley biomedical-health publication)
"A symposium sponsored by the Perinatal Biology and
Infant Mortality Branch, National Institute of Child
Health and Human Development, Stanford, California,
December 6-9, 1970."
1. Maternal and infant welfare—Congresses.
2. Pregnancy—Congresses. I. Kretchmer, Norman,
1923–   ed. II. Hasselmeyer, Eileen G., ed.
III. United States. National Institute of Child
Health and Human Development. Perinatal Biology and
Infant Mortality Branch. [DNLM: 1. Fetal diseases—
Congresses. 2. Infant, Newborn, Disease—Congresses.
2. Infant mortality—Congresses. 3. Pregnancy
complications—Congresses. WS420 H811 1973]
RG940.H67   618.2'4   73-14803
ISBN 0-471-50723-7

FOREWORD

Research activities in perinatal biology represent one of the major concerns of the National Institute of Child Health and Human Development.

I am pleased that so many of the nation's authorities were able to assemble to discuss their present investigative activities as well as directions for future research. The results of these investigations will be important to the well-being of mothers, infants, and children throughout the world.

Perinatal biology is particularly demanding, since the concept of the mother and fetus as a biological unit complicates research and also requires unique training experiences for investigators. However, by approaching the problems of the health of both individuals as a unit, we are more likely to obtain new knowledge that will lead to even greater reduction of infant and maternal mobidity and mortality.

I believe this conference can influence the entire field of child health and human development by pointing the way to future achievements in research.

Director
National Institute of Child Health
and Human Development

GERALD D. LAVECK, M.D.

PREFACE

There have been a number of conferences held during the past few years concerned with problems of the infant. These meetings were, in general, designed to respond to an immediate concern for the infant-at-risk. This particular symposium was constructed to respond to the need for a review of potentialities for research in the area of perinatal biology. The concern, here, is not only for the infant but also for the mother. Hopefully, we have created more questions than we have answered. These questions should serve as a basis for future investigation.

The makeup of the planning committee reflects this medical multidisciplinary approach. This committee consisted of Drs. Edward Quilligan, James Metcalfe, Sydney Segal, Joseph Dancis, Eileen Hasselmeyer, and Norman Kretchmer. Each of these scientists represents a completely different field in perinatal biology. Consequently, each served as a moderator of a session that most closely represented his scientific acumen.

The emphasis in this conference is research, particularly in regard to potential cross-disciplinary approaches, and ranges from molecular biology to epidemiology. Research is the foundation for training and patient care. It would be redundant to extoll the virtues of each of these fields as being separate, since they are continually interdependent. The conference also moves between these three categories, with a constant emphasis on those areas where there are potentialities for unearthing new knowledge.

The need for the conference evolved from concerns of the staff of the Perinatal Biology and Infant Mortality Program of the National Institute of Child Health and Human Development in the development of program activities aimed at assisting the support of scientific investigations. It is anticipated that this knowledge will result both in the achievement of maximum health and well-being for every pregnant woman and her progeny and the lowering of the infant mortality rate in this nation. Also, it is important to strengthen scientific and communication ties between the health professions responsible for care of mother and infant, and to identify manpower needs necessary to advance delivery of health care and research in the perinatal period.

Although the conference was informal, with a great deal of latitude for free and candid discussion, this report is presented in a more organized fashion so as to increase facility for the reader.

Probably the most important general conclusion reached by all participants was that if our knowledge and manpower in the all important field of perinatal biology is to advance, then the unionistic separation between pediatrics and obstetrics must disappear.

Stanford University   NORMAN KRETCHMER, M.D., Ph.D.

National Institute of Child Health   EILEEN G. HASSELMEYER, Ph.D., R.N.
and Human Development

PARTICIPANTS

CHARLES A. ALFORD, M.D.
Meyer Professor of Pediatric Research
Department of Pediatrics
University of Alabama School of Medicine
Birmingham, Alabama 35233
(Perinatology, Infectious Disease)

ROBERT H. ALWAY, M.D.
Professor
Department of Pediatrics
Stanford University Medical Center
Stanford, California 94305
(Maternal and Child Health)

SIR DUGALD BAIRD
Belding Scholar ACCC
Emeritus Professor of Obstetrics and Gynaecology
Department of Medical Sociology Research Unit
University of Aberdeen
Aberdeen, Scotland
(Maternal and Child Health)

HENRY L. BARNETT, M.D.
Professor and Chairman
Department of Pediatrics
Albert Einstein College of Medicine
Bronx, New York 10461
(Developmental Renal Physiology)

RICHARD BEHRMAN, M.D.
Professor and Chairman
Department of Pediatrics
College of Physicians and Surgeons
Columbia University
New York, New York 10032
(Fetal and Newborn Physiology)

JOSEPH DANCIS, M.D.*
Professor
Department of Pediatrics
New York University Medical Center
New York, New York 10016
(Placental Physiology, Biochemical Genetics)

SANFORD DORNBUSCH, Ph.D.
Professor
Department of Sociology
Stanford University
Stanford, California 94305
(Sociology, Human Biology)

JEAN GOODWIN, B.A.
Harvard Medical School
Class of '71
Boston, Massachusetts 02115
(Maternal Health)

HARRY H. GORDON, M.D.
Professor
Department of Pediatrics
Yeshiva University
Bronx, New York 10461
(Human Developmental Biology)

WILLIAM W. GREULICH, Ph.D.
Research Biologist
Departments of Anatomy and Pediatrics
Stanford University Medical Center
Stanford, California 94305
(Physical Anthropology)

EILEEN G. HASSELMEYER, Ph.D., R.N *†
Director
Perinatal Biology and Infant Mortality Branch
National Institute of Child Health and Human Development
Bethesda, Maryland 20014
(Perinatal Biology and Nursing Science)

ANDRE E. HELLEGERS, M.D.
Professor of Obstetrics-Gynecology and Physiology-Biophysics
Department of Obstetrics and Gynecology
Georgetown University
Washington, D.C. 20007
(Fetal and Placental Physiology)

LOUIS M. HELLMAN, M.D.
Deputy Assistant Secretary for Population Affairs
Department of Health, Education, and Welfare
Washington, D.C. 20201
(Administration, Reproductive Biology)

CHARLES H. HENDRICKS, M.D.
Professor and Chairman
Department of Obstetrics and Gynecology
University of North Carolina School of Medicine
Chapel Hill, North Carolina 27514
(Reproductive Biology)

JOSEPH C. HWANG, Ph.D.
Health Scientist Administrator
Perinatal Biology and Infant Mortality
National Institute of Child Health and Human Development
Bethesda, Maryland 20014
(Fetal Health and Development)

M. HARRY JENNISON, M.D.
Medical Director, Children's Hospital at Stanford and
Clinical Professor, Department of Pediatrics
Stanford University Medical Center
Stanford, California 94305
(Child Health Care)

IRWIN H. KAISER, M.D., Ph.D.
Professor
Department of Gynecology and Obstetrics
Albert Einstein College of Medicine
Bronx, New York 10461
(Reproductive Physiology, Maternal Health)

EDWARD KASS, M.D., Ph.D.
Professor
Department of Medicine
Harvard University Medical School
Boston, Massachusetts 02118
(Infectious Disease, Epidemiology)

NORMAN KRETCHMER, M.D., Ph.D.*†
Professor
Department of Pediatrics
Stanford University Medical Center
Stanford, California 94305
(Developmental Biochemistry, Perinatal Growth)

JAN LANGMAN, M.D., Ph.D.
Professor and Chairman
Department of Anatomy
University of Virginia
Charlottesville, Virginia 22901
(Embryology)

LAWRENCE D. LONGO, M.D.
Professor of Physiology and Obstetrics and Gynecology
Department of Obstetrics and Gynecology
Loma Linda University
Loma Linda, California 92354
(Reproductive Biology)

CHARLES E. McLENNAN, M.D.
Professor and Chairman
Department of Gynecology and Obstetrics
Stanford University Medical Center
Stanford, California 94305
(Reproductive Physiology, Pathology)

JAMES METCALFE, M.D.*
Professor
Department of Medicine
University of Oregon Medical School
Portland, Oregon 97201
(Placental Physiology)

JAMES MILLER, M.D.
Professor and Head, Division of Medical Genetics
University of British Columbia
Vancouver 9, B.C., Canada
(Teratology)

ORLANDO J. MILLER, M.D.
Professor
Department of Obstetrics and Gynecology
and Human Genetics and Development
Columbia University
New York, New York 10032
(Cytogenetics, Teratology)

ALEXANDER MINKOWSKI, M.D.
Professor and Chief
Neonatal Research Unit
Clinique Baudeloque
Paris, France
(Neonatology)

EDWARD QUILLIGAN, M.D.*
Professor and Chairman
Department of Obstetrics-Gynecology
University of Southern California Medical School
Los Angeles, California 90033
(Fetal Physiology)

O. RANSOME-KUTI, M.B., F.R.C.P.
Professor
Department of Pediatrics
University College Hospital
University of Lagos, Nigeria
(Pediatric Medicine and Child Health)

LEON ROSENBERG, M.D.
Professor
Department of Genetics
Yale University
New Haven, Connecticut 06510
(Human Biochemical Genetics)

ETTORE ROSSI, M.D.
Professor and Head
Department of Pediatrics
Kinderspital-University of Bern
Bern, Switzerland
(Pediatrics, Carbohydrate Metabolism)

HERBERT C. SCHWARTZ, M.D.
Professor and Chairman
Department of Pediatrics
Stanford University Medical Center
Stanford, California 94305
(Hematology)

SYDNEY SEGAL, M.D.*
Professor
Department of Pediatrics
University of British Columbia
Vancouver 9, B.C., Canada
(Neonatology, Respiratory Physiology)

FABIO SERENI, M.D.
Professor
Department of Pediatrics
University of Milan
Milan, Italy
(Developmental Biochemistry)

JANE SHOWACRE, Ph.D.
Biologist
Perinatal Biology and Infant Mortality Branch
National Institute of Child Health and Human Development
Bethesda, Maryland 20014
(Developmental Biology)

WILLIAM SILVERMAN, M.D.
Chief, Perinatology Section
Kaiser Foundation Hospital
San Francisco, California 94115
(Perinatology)

PHILIP SUNSHINE, M.D.
Associate Professor
Department of Pediatrics
Stanford University Medical Center
Stanford, California 94305
(Neonatology, Gastroenterology)

GILBERT WOODSIDE, Ph.D.
Associate Director, Extramural Programs
National Institute of Child Health and Human Development
Bethesda, Maryland 20014
(Administration, Developmental Biology)

CONTENTS

Horizons in
Perinatal Research
IMPLICATIONS FOR CLINICAL CARE

Scope of the Problem

Some Clouds
Over the Horizons
of Perinatal Biology

Harry H. Gordon

John Gardner, in acknowledging an Albert Einstein Commemorative Award in May 1969, ended his brief remarks with three pithy sentences which I remember essentially as follows: "These are difficult times. One of the most difficult things is to look honestly at oneself and one's own activities. Be of courage."

I should like to address myself to a hard look at our own activities. How is it that with all the improvements in medical therapy that have stemmed from research,[6] we find ourselves out of favor with the citizenry? A major complaint of the American citizenry is the inability to find medical care. The rich cannot find it as promptly as they find answers to their other felt needs. The middle class finds the increasing costs unreasonable and the services inadequate even with the help of insurance plans. Many of the poor, whose expectations have been stimulated by television, the civil rights movement and the programs of the Office of Economic Opportunity, receive substandard care whether in the city slums or rural backwoods.

Eli Ginzberg, human resources economist and logistics expert for the Surgeon General of the U.S. Army during World War II, says that doubling the

number of physicians will not substantially improve medical care unless we
redistribute their services.[2] Sidney Garfield says that a National Health
Insurance plan is not enough and that we must reorganize the system of care and
give to trained paramedical personnel the responsibility for health services to a
greater proportion of the populace.[1]

If we wish to continue with research and teaching activities, which are part
of the life blood of medical care, it is not enough that these be satisfying both
intellectually and emotionally to us personally, in addition to being socially
useful. We have to convince a skeptical public of the inherent value of both
laboratory research and clinical research and teaching.[3] This is not a job only for
public relations experts or information specialists. First, we practicing
physicians, institutional or private, must match our socially minded medical
students in concern for studying and delivering improved health services to all
people. Julius Richmond asserts that academicians as well as practitioners, either
as individuals or through their organizations, can take little credit for their
activities in this regard in the 40 years since publication of the Wilbur report on
medical care in the United States.[7]

Second, we must educate the public on the value of laboratory and clinical
research, teaching and training to clinical medicine and we must do this without
promising unrealistic crash programs. I am proud that we never promised the
Kennedy Foundation a crash program for prevention and cure of mental
retardation at the time of the construction grant to help the Albert Einstein
College of Medicine match the National Institutes of Health grants. Rather, we
went along with Pope John who quoted an old Italian folk saying, "He who goes
slowly, goes far and arrives safely," and with Rabbi Tarfon who said 1900 years
ago, "It is not for thee to finish the work, but neither art thou free to desist
from it," and with President Kennedy's inaugural injunction: "But let us begin."

During the past decades, our academic promotion committees have not
recognized excellence in teaching and patient care. Clinicians and teachers have
suffered from these insults, but I believe they magnified them. Mrs. Franklin
Roosevelt said that no one could snub her, and I wish clinicians and teachers
would not be so defensive. After all, in their hypothalami, they experience daily
satisfactions from students they have helped develop, and from patients and
their families whose anxieties they have diminished, sometimes even by the cure
of the disease. What worries me now is that with a long overdue philosophical
swing, and with inadequate money available for support of medical care and
medical education, teachers and clinicians will turn on the research scientists,
not recognizing that research advances are what we have to transmit to improve
the quality of patient care. The clinician has an important role in teaching the
citizenry the importance of research and teaching. Dr. Barnaby Keeney, retired
Professor of History and President of Brown University, spoke to the National
Academy of Sciences on "The Bridge of Values."[4] In reading Dr. Keeney's
address, I thought at first that his discussion of a bridge of values between

science and the humanities did not have much to do with this conference because all of us think of ourselves as scientists. But science, which is one expression of human potential, is supposed to be in the service of people just as religion and music and literature are.

If this is true, one of the main clouds on the horizons of research is the divisiveness which has developed between laboratory scientist and clinical scientist, and between teacher and practitioner, which threatens the quality and quantity of the goods we deliver conjointly to the public. I plead, therefore, for understanding of personal differences[5] and binding up of the wounds that have developed over the years. It is destructive to attack "Flexnerism" in order to push "primary physicianship." I want them both combined in our medical schools so that some young people can opt for one, the other, or be willing to serve as bridge persons.

I would like to close with a mixture of anecdote, maxim and quote. The late Dr. Edwards Park, when he was still a vigorous 75 years old, was watching a female guest at his home, probably not too far behind him in years, laying bricks in the patio. "I would help you," said he, "if I weren't retired." And though I'm not quite on the shelf yet, I am usually only keynote speaker with narrative rather than "hard" data; I don't have even a twinge of guilt in quoting a maximum that used to be in Dr. Sidney Colowick's office in the Department of Biology at Johns Hopkins: "Ye of faint heart, remember this, nothing is impossible to the man who doesn't have to do it himself." And I don't feel guilty, though I am being hortatory, when I quote to laboratory scientists and clinicians and teachers and practitioners the words of Hillel, a rabbinic sage who lived 2,000 years ago: "If I am not for myself, who will be for me? But if I am for myself alone, what am I?" So go about your work, but go about it consciously in the service of man.

BIBLIOGRAPHY

1. Garfield, S. R., "The Delivery of Medical Care." Scientific American, 222:15, Number 4, April, 1969.

2. Ginzberg, E. and Ostow, M., *Men, Money and Medicine.* Columbia University Press, New York and London, 1969.

3. Gordon, H. H., "Some Observations on Contributions of Biomedical Research to Maternal and Child Health," presented at the symposium on "Research in the Service of Man—An Inquiry into Public Policy on Biomedical Knowledge: Research, Development and Use" (Government Printing Office), Oklahoma City, Oklahoma, October 24-27, 1966.

4. 5. Keeney, B., "The Bridge of Values," Sci., 169:26, 1970.

5. Kubie, L. S., "Some Unsolved Problems of the Scientific Career," Am. Sci. 41:596 (1953), and 42:104 (1954).

6. The Life Sciences, Committee on Research in the Life Sciences of the Committee on Science and Public Policy, National Academy of Sciences, Washington, D.C., 1970.

7. Richmond, J. B., *Currents in American Medicine—A Developmental View of Medical Care and Education,* Harvard University Press, Cambridge, Massachusetts, 1969.

Environmental Influences on Maternal and Infant Capabilities

Introduction

Edward Quilligan

The final product of conception is the result of interaction between two general biological phenomena, genetic inheritance and the environment in which the conceptus grows. The environment of the fetus, like that of the adult, is modified by factors beyond that individual's control. Fetal growth is related to the adequacy of maternal nutrition in the animal model and in the human. Even though the fetus can seemingly grow at the expense of the maternal organism, the fetus as well as the mother pays a price. The question "how high the price" needs an answer. Is the price that the fetus pays simply life or death, or are there long-term effects that reflect on the next generation in terms of a high fetal risk. Some of the studies we will hear about and discuss this morning will direct themselves to these fundamental questions.

Sociological Considerations of Maternal and Infant Capabilities

Sir Dugald Baird

The outcome of pregnancy is influenced by genetic factors, the mother's age, the number of previous pregnancies, her level of health and physique, and by the standard of obstetric and paediatric care available to her.

In Britain, the introduction of the National Health Service in 1948 made it possible to organize a comprehensive area Maternity Service in each region of the country based on specialist hospitals. The responsibility of the hospital and of the specialist staff was widened from the treatment of the individual patients under their immediate care to the provision of a service for all expectant mothers in the area. In Scotland, the responsibility for the planning and running of each defined region was the responsibility of a Regional Hospital Board, and in Scotland it was also responsible for the provision of clinical facilities for teaching medical students. The teaching staff of the hospitals, in turn, played an integral part in the provision of specialist care for all women in the region. It, therefore, became possible to organize a uniformly high standard of care for all.

In Aberdeen, in 1948 all expectant mothers were given the opportunity of a hospital confinement and 85 percent availed themselves of this offer. The remaining 15 percent were mostly women of high parity from the semi- and unskilled classes who had been accustomed to home confinement and were unwilling to come to the hospital, although many were "high risk" cases. The domiciliary service was provided by the Local Health Authority. All obstetric records, irrespective of the place of confinement, were stored in the central maternity hospital and thus were easily available for study and analysis. From 1948 onwards, complete obstetric records for the city were compiled. It was, therefore, possible to assess results of treatment, and study the effects of the environment from which the women came on their reproductive efficiency. In addition, the hospital staff were organized as a single division of obstetrics.

Efficient organization of services was possibly easier in the smaller regions and Figure 1 shows that the perinatal mortality rate in the city of Aberdeen in the North-East Region of Scotland, and Dundee in the East Region (each with a population of 200,000) fell more quickly than in Edinburgh in the South-East Region and in Glasgow in the South-West Region, with populations of 500,000 and 1,000,000 respectively.

The recipe for easy and efficient childbearing is simple and little more than common sense, viz. first pregnancy soon after maturity (say between the ages of 18 and 22), a high standard of health and physique, cessation of childbearing by the age of 30, and restriction of the total number to not more than four. In the 1930's, primigravidae in the semi- and unskilled social classes in Britain were young but often badly grown and malnourished, had too many children, and sometimes continued childbearing to the age of 40 or over. Women in the professional and managerial classes (The Registrar General's Social Classes I and II) were often too old when they had their first child, but usually had the advantage of being well grown, well nourished, and well educated. Table I taken from the first report of the National Birthday Trust, Perinatal Mortality Survey of 1958, published in 1963, shows the height of the mother, the standard of education, and the perinatal mortality ratio (the ratio for all women having a value of 100), in relation to the social class of the woman's father and that of her husband. The women whose fathers and husbands are professional men are taller than those in any other group. A higher percentage of them have had more than the minimum amount of education, and they have the lowest perinatal mortality ratio (71). The assumption is that as a group they have been reared in the best environment and are, therefore, most likely to have grown to their genetically determined height and to have received the best standard of care and of education. They are likely, therefore, to plan their marriage and childbearing better than other groups. Those who move up in the social scale on marriage are taller and have lower perinatal ratios than those who do not rise or move down. If one equates for age, the perinatal mortality rate in primigravidae from Social Classes I and II is only half that in primigravidae from Social Classes IV and V in each individual cause group.

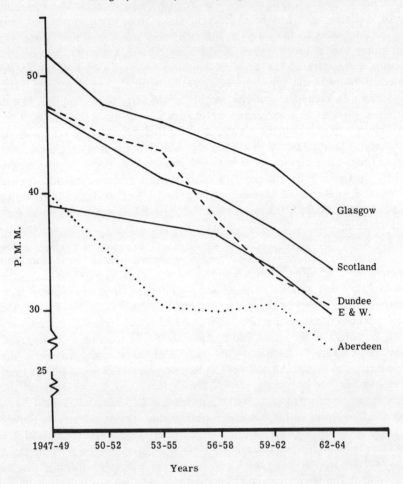

PERINATAL MORTALITY 1947-64

Glasgow, Scotland, Dundee, England & Wales, Aberdeen.

Fig. 1

TABLE I. Height of Wives, Educational Standard and Mortality Ratio
(all parities) by Socio-Economic Group of Father and Husband
(National Birthday Trust Mortality Survey 1958)

Husband's Socio-Economic Group	Father's Socio-economic Group											
	Professional			Nonmanual			Skilled			Unskilled		
	(a)	(b)	(c)	(a)	(b)	(c)	(a)	(b)	(c)	(a)	(b)	(c)
Professional	46	84	(71)	40	71	(72)	37	47	(76)	32	39	(93)
Nonmanual	43	73	(76)	36	44	(85)	30	30	(83)	26	18	(89)
Skilled	34	48	(81)	32	32	(89)	28	17	(94)	23	11	(104)
Unskilled	27	42	(117)	28	20	(82)	26	12	(102)	24	10	(124)
All	41	69	(79)	34	43	(85)	29	21	(91)	25	12	(111)

(a) % 65" or more in height
(b) % Educated beyond the minimum
(c) Mortality ratio

Table II shows the incidence of babies weighing 2500 g or less in 9154 Aberdeen primigravidae in the years 1958-67. It shows that the incidence of low weight babies increases with decreasing height of the mother. In gestations of 38 weeks or more, there is no social class difference in the percentage of low weight babies in women of the same height, but in gestations of less than 38 weeks, the percentage of low weight babies increases both with decreasing social status and decreasing height of the mother, the extremes being 2.2 percent in tall women from Social Classes I to IIIa (nonmanual social classes) and 5.7 percent in short women in Social Classes IV and V.

TABLE II. Incidence of Babies Weighing 2500 g or Less in
9154 Primiparae in Aberdeen 1958–67 by Social Class
and Height of Mother and Length of Gestation

Social Class	T (64")		M		S (61")		All heights	
	<37.	38-	<37	38-	<37	38-	<37	38-
I - IIIA	2.2	1.9	3.3	3.8	4.8	5.5	3.1	3.3
IIIB & C	3.1	1.8	3.5	3.0	5.1	4.1	3.9	3.0
IV & V	3.6	1.5	4.6	4.4	5.7	4.5	5.0	4.0
All Classes	3.0	1.8	4.0	3.6	5.3	4.6	3.9	3.3
Numbers	2643		4521		1990		9154	

One may conclude, therefore, that the benefit derived from a good environment in childhood is not confined to optimum growth of the skeleton but affects the growth and development of all organs of the body necessary for efficient childbearing.

The Influence of National Events
on Perinatal Mortality Rates

The relationship between national events and the perinatal mortality rates in Britain since 1928 helps to throw some light on the influence of social circumstances on childbearing. The sequence of events can be summarized as follows:

Early 1930's	Economic depression	Slight rise in P.N.M. rate
1936-1940	Fall in unemployment	Slight fall in P.N.M. rate
1940-1947	War condition	Slight fall in P.N.M. rate
1948-1957	Postwar period and first 10 years of NHS	Slight fall in P.N.M. rate
1957-1969	Welfare state, full employment and early marriage	Steady and substantial fall in P.N.M. rates

The fall in the rate during the war was surprising. It was greatest in South Wales where unemployment and the prewar perinatal mortality rates were highest. It was least in London and the South-East of England where the prewar perinatal mortality and unemployment rates were lowest. The wartime fall was thought to demonstrate the beneficial effect of a good diet during pregnancy in women who had been chronically undernourished for many years. The Government's policy was to give priority for essential foods to expectant mothers and young children accompanied by excellent publicity and education on the importance of good nutrition. The stark reality of the situation and the will to survive were also important factors making for full cooperation by the public. The limit to what could be done by improving the diet during pregnancy on a national scale had probably been reached by 1948. The very slight reduction in the perinatal mortality rate in the first 10 years of the National Health Service was disappointing but scarcely surprising when one considers the disruption of medical services during the war and the fact that even before the war the maternity services were inadequate and badly organized. Hospital beds were too few in number, and the training of medical students in practical obstetrics was very deficient. Figure 2 shows that in 1957, there were still considerable regional differences in the perinatal mortality rate. The rate was highest in the industrial North and in South Wales and lowest in London and the South-East of England. The Perinatal Mortality Survey organized by the National Birthday Trust in 1958 studied the causes of the perinatal deaths and the reasons for these geographical differences. The definitions of causes of perinatal mortality which were used in the survey are contained in "Perinatal

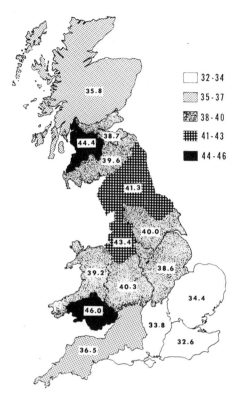

Fig. 2. Perinatal mortality rate, England, Wales, and Scotland, 1957.

Problems" (1969), the second volume of the official report. They were divided into an "environmental" and an "obstetric" group of causes. The main components of the "environmental" cause group were malformations of the central nervous system and "unexplained prematurity." Deaths in the latter category occur in babies weighing less than 2500 g (usually much less) where no well-established obstetric complication coexisted. In other words, no clear predisposing clinical cause can be found from both causes. Death rates are higher in the semi- and unskilled manual classes (Social Classes IV and V). Deaths in the "obstetric" cause group were associated with difficult labour, preeclampsia, unexplained death of a baby weighing more than 2500 g occurring before, during, or soon after labour, or with rhesus incompatibility. The United Kingdom was divided into three zones: North, Central, and South. The perinatal mortality rate was found to increase from South to North very largely in the "environmental" group of causes. In each zone the death rate from "environmental" causes was greater in urban than rural areas, while the death rate in the "obstetric" cause group was higher in rural areas. Women were tallest in the South and shortest in the North and in each zone taller in the rural than the urban areas. The conclusions drawn were that the higher perinatal mortality rates in the North compared to the South were the result mainly of the poorer health and physique of mothers in the North, especially in the overcrowded slums of the large industrial cities. The higher death rate from "obstetric" causes in rural areas, despite the fact that the women were taller and healthier, pointed to the need for easier access to skilled obstetric care in the rural areas.

With regard to prevention of deaths in the "environmental" cause group, it was noted that those associated with unexplained prematurity or low birth weight fell substantially during the war, but those from central nervous system malformations did not, suggesting that improved nutrition during pregnancy, in the context in which it occurred in wartime Britain, was not sufficient to lessen the risk of anencephaly. Another explanation might be that since the neural canal closes very early in pregnancy, even before the pregnancy is diagnosed with certainty, any improved intake of food during pregnancy would occur too late.

The possible effect of migration must be considered in studying geographical differences in perinatal mortality rates. For many years in Britain there has been considerable migration from North to South and from the depressed to the affluent areas. Migrants were taller and had lower perinatal mortality rates than those in the same social class who did not migrate. While this may not affect the perinatal mortality rate in the area to which the migrants went, it does have the indirect effect of raising the rate in the area from which they came or at least in delaying a reduction in the death rate.

Figure 3 shows that in the years 1948-57, when the perinatal mortality rate in England and Wales remained stationary, the rate in Aberdeen continued to fall, because, as already stated, 85 percent of the deliveries from 1948 onwards took place in the teaching hospitals under the care of specialists. By 1960, there remained little scope for reducing the perinatal mortality rate in Aberdeen with the clinical "material" available so long as the women with large families continued to have their babies at home. However, the drift to hospital by the women in this "high risk" group began in 1960 and was completed by 1968. Meanwhile, in the years 1958-62, the perinatal mortality rate in the city rose due to an increase in the death rate from central nervous system malformations. This started in 1951 in young primigravidae from Social Classes IV and V, and within a few years affected older primigravidae from the other social classes and multiparae in all social classes.

Table IIIa shows that the stillbirth rate from anencephaly in Scotland rose in first pregnancies from 2.2 per 1000 births in 1948-50 to 3.5 in 1951-53, in second pregnancies from 1.7 per 1000 in 1951-53 to 2.3 in 1954-57, and in third pregnancies from 2.0 in 1951-53 to 2.9 in 1954-57. In fourth and subsequent pregnancies the rate was high (over 3 per 1000) between 1939 and 1965, with a slightly higher rate from 1954 onwards. Table IIIb shows that in women under the age of 25 the stillbirth rate from anencephaly (already high in the 15-19 age group) rose in 1951-53, whereas in those over the age of 25 most of the rise in the death rate occurred in the years 1954-61. The younger age groups contained

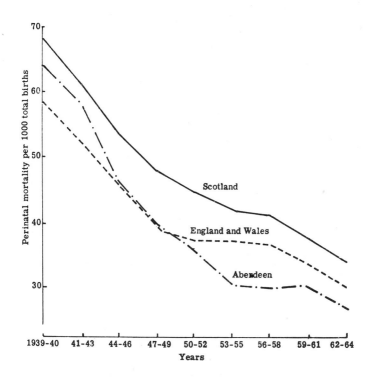

Fig. 3. Perinatal mortality rates in England and Wales, Scotland, and Aberdeen, 1939-40 to 1962-64. Reprinted, by permission, from Butler, N.R. and Alberman, E.D. (eds.): *Perinatal Problems,* Edinburgh and London, E. and S. Livingstone, Ltd., 1969, p. 256.

TABLE III. Stillbirth Rate from Anencephaly
Scotland in Three Year Age Groups
1939-68

(a) By Number of Pregnancy

Preg-nancy	1939-41	1942-44	1945-47	1948-50	1951-53	1954-57	1958-61	1962-65	1966-68
1st	2.0	2.6	2.5	2.2	3.5	3.0	3.7	3.0	2.8
2nd	1.7	2.3	1.8	1.8	1.7	2.3	2.4	2.4	1.5
3rd	2.8	2.4	2.4	2.5	2.0	2.9	3.2	2.6	2.0
4th	3.4	3.0	2.5	3.0	3.1	3.4	3.1	3.4	2.2
5th	3.8	3.6	3.3	3.4	3.6	3.8	4.2	3.7	3.3
All preg.	2.5	2.7	2.6	2.3	2.7	2.9	3.2	2.9	2.2

(b) By Age of Mother

Age	1939-41	1942-44	1945-47	1948-50	1951-53	1954-57	1958-61	1962-65	1966-68
15-19	2.6	2.4	2.9	3.2	3.8	3.9	3.8	3.3	2.7
20-24	1.9	2.5	2.1	2.2	2.8	2.9	3.0	2.9	2.2
25-28	2.1	2.4	2.4	1.9	2.4	2.4	2.9	2.5	2.0
30-34	2.4	2.9	2.3	2.3	2.4	2.9	3.2	2.7	2.2
35+	3.4	3.0	2.9	2.8	3.2	3.5	3.7	3.1	2.9
All ages	2.4	2.6	2.5	2.3	2.7	3.0	3.1	2.7	2.3

a high proportion of primigravidae from Social Classes IV and V and the older age groups contained primigravidae from the upper social classes and multiparae from all social classes. Analysis of the data by the year of birth of the mother shows that many more than expected were born between the years 1928 and 1932, at the time when the industrial depression was at its worst and unemployment in Scotland reached almost 30 percent. Not surprisingly, the first rise in the stillbirth rate from anencephaly occurred in young women aged 18-20 from the lowest social classes, because they were particularly vulnerable. The second peak in the death rate in 1958-61 is related to a rise in the occurrence of anencephaly in women in the other social classes who are up to five years older: for example, in the 25-29 and 30-34 age groups in the years 1954-57 and 1958-61 respectively. Again, the upper social classes having more resources would be able to protect themselves and their children from the effects of the depression for a time at least and would be quickest to recover when conditions began to improve. Hence, the short duration of the rise in the stillbirth rate from anencephaly in Social Classes I and II (between 1958 and 1961). At the opposite end of the social scale it will be seen [Table IIIa] that the death rate in 5th+ pregnancies was high (3.8 per 1000) in 1939-41 and rose to 4.2 per 1000 in 1958-61, and during 1962-65 was still as high as 3.3 per 1000. However, it will be seen that in the years 1966-68, the stillbirth rate from anencephaly for all pregnancies has now fallen below the 1939-41 figure. This holds for each pregnancy, suggesting that a substantial decrease in the death rate is likely.

Dr. Ingalls subjected mice with a tendency to produce an occasional anencephalic offspring to oxygen lack at a critical stage of pregnancy by altering the atmospheric pressure of the air they breathed. This produced a marked increase in the percentage of anencephalic mice born. In mice with a tendency to produce offspring with exomphalos, oxygen lack causes an increased incidence of malformations of this type. The changes in the environment therefore produced an excess in the type of malformation normally produced. The type of change in the environment was less important than the stage in pregnancy at which it operated.

The fall in the stillbirth rate during the 1939-45 war was thought to be due largely to improvements in diets of mothers during pregnancy, particularly in areas of high unemployment where stillbirth rates were highest. There was no decline in the stillbirth rate from malformations of the central nervous system. This might be because the neural canal closes very early in pregnancy so that the damage was done before the mother had time to improve her diet.

The epidemiology of the increase in the stillbirth rate from anencephaly in Scotland from 1951 onwards suggests that damage was done to the future mother early in childhood or before birth as a result of extreme poverty and malnutrition in the family of origin. How this would act, however, is not clear. The incidence of anencephaly in Social Class I is approximately 0.5 per 1000 and in Social Class V (the unskilled manual class) is between 4 and 5 per 1000, suggesting that the unfavourable environment increases the incidence by about 10 times. The rise in the stillbirth rate from anencephaly lasted for about 15 years (1951-65) in Social Class V and for only three years in Social Class I, probably because of the greater resources of those in the professional classes.

The high stillbirth rates from anencephaly in Ireland has been attributed to ethnic factors, but it could be the result of poverty. Rates are high in Liverpool and Glasgow, both of which cities have a large Irish immigrant population. Many of these are in the semi- and unskilled manual classes so that it would be very difficult to disentangle ethnic factors from those of poverty.

The almost complete absence of anencephaly in many parts of Africa and in the South Pacific area, for example Malaya, Borneo, and Hong Kong, among people with very low standards of living, suggests ethnic differences. In Britain, the combination of a tendency to anencephaly plus overcrowding, unbalanced diet, cold damp climate, air pollution, and a lack of sunshine may all help to produce the very high death rate of CNS malformations. How far this is the direct result of conditions during the pregnancy and how far a more indirect effect acting through damage to the mother at the time of her own birth is not clear. In Scotland, the sequence of events from 1951 onwards suggests that the rise in the stillbirth rate from anencephaly between 1951 and 1965 was related to damage to the mother at the time of her birth.

The probable explanation of the stationary perinatal mortality rate in England and Wales between 1948-57 is that the improvement brought about by better obstetrics was neutralized by the rise in the perinatal death rate from CNS malformations. This rise in the death rate occurred in all other CNS malformations as well as in anencephaly. Many more of these deaths occurred in the first seven days of life. In the case of Aberdeen, the fall in the perinatal mortality rate from obstetric causes was large enough to maintain the fall in the overall perinatal mortality rate till 1957, but, here again, the downward trend was halted and, in fact, it was reversed slightly because very few avoidable deaths still occurred.

In Scotland, the stillbirth rate from anencephaly varies from 0.5 per 1000 births in Social Class I to between 4 and 5 per 1000 in Social Class V. Thus, it seems that in Caucasians in Scotland the most unfavourable environment can increase the incidence by up to 10 times that found in the most favourable environment. There are, however, ethnic differences in incidence. For example, anencephaly is very rare in West Africans, but West Africans who have lived in the United States for generations have a higher incidence than those living in West Africa but much lower than Caucasians living in affluent areas in the United States. The increase in anencephaly in the descendants of the original African immigrants is thought to be a measure of the degree of mixing of West Africans and Caucasians. According to Reed (1969), using the Fe^a gene of the Duffy group, which is almost absent in West Africans and has a frequency of 43 percent in white Americans, the white mixture in West Africans is 19 percent.

A relationship between malformations and a variety of agents given to the mother at a critical time in early pregnancy is well known in animals and the teratogenic effect of thalidomide and rubella are also well established, but it is difficult to explain the epidemiological findings just described in this way or the steep social gradient in anencephaly which is so obvious in Scotland and Northern Ireland. It seems possible that damage may be done to the future mother early in childhood or even before birth as a result of extreme poverty and malnutrition in the family of origin. The manner in which this unfavourable environment affects the reproductive efficiency 20 years later is not certain. Is it through damage to vital tissues or mechanisms necessary for reproduction later, or is it because of a carry-over of a way of life from the previous generation whereby the foetus in the next generation is also subjected to the same "malnutrition" during its intrauterine growth?

The very satisfactory decline in the perinatal mortality rate which has occurred in Britain since 1957 seems to have two main causes. First, the steady improvement in the standards of obstetric care brought about by a better organization of the maternity and paediatric services throughout the country, more consultants more strategically placed, more maternity beds, better training of obstetric specialists, and more well trained general practitioner obstetricians; secondly, the much improved health and physique of mothers born about the end of the 1939-45 war who now make up the majority of childbearing women in Britain today. The earlier age at which childbearing starts is an advantage obstetrically and is an index of full employment and more affluence. More efficient family planning has resulted in smaller families and, finally, the fact that the women born in the worst years of the industrial depression, who had high perinatal death rates from all causes, have now completed their childbearing.

Nevertheless, we still have in our midst many casualties of the living conditions brought about by the industrial revolution. This change from an agrarian society increased Britain's wealth and power in the world, but too little attention was given to the health and happiness of those who worked in the mines and the factories. Consequently, there are still areas, especially in some of the large cities, where living conditions are still bad and perinatal death rates from "environmental" causes are high.

The situation in Scandinavia presents a striking contrast. Sweden is the best example of a small country which has become prosperous and at the same time adopted a progressive social policy which raised the health and physique to a high level in all sections of society. Table IV shows that in 1961-63 the perinatal mortality rate in Sweden was 12 per 1000. In the Netherlands, the rate

TABLE IV. Perinatal Mortality Rates 1961-63

Country	Stillbirth Rate	Death Rate 0-6 Days	Perinatal Mortality Rate
Sweden	10.0	8.9	18.9
Netherlands	13.1	10.1	23.2
England & Wales	15.3	11.0	26.3
Scotland	16.2	13.0	29.2

was 23. The stillbirth rate is the better measure of the standard of obstetric care, and the first week death rate the better measure of the health of the population at risk (because of the great importance of deaths in babies weighing less than 2500 g as a cause of death and its association with poor social circumstances). Since the difference between these two countries is greater in the stillbirth than the first week death rate, it seems probable that the higher perinatal mortality in the Netherlands is associated mostly with the low incidence of hospital delivery. Certain of the prosperous areas in Britain have perinatal mortality rates approaching that of Sweden, but for much of Britain a high death rate from CNS malformations and "unexplained prematurity" keeps the national stillbirth and first week death rates high.

BIBLIOGRAPHY

1. Butler, N.R. and Alberman, E.D. (eds.), *Perinatal Problems: Second Report of the 1958 British Perinatal Mortality Survey,* Edinburgh and London, E. and S. Livingstone, Ltd., 1963, pp. 392.

2. Butler, N.R. and Bonham, D.G., *Perinatal Mortality: First Report of the 1958 British Perinatal Mortality Survey,* Edinburgh and London, E. and S. Livingstone, Ltd., 1963.

3. "Foetal Mortality (1961/63): According to cause per 100,000 live births," *WHO Epidem. Vital Statist. Rep. No. 6:* 257, 1966.

Sociological Considerations of Maternal and Infant Capabilities

Discussion

Sanford Dornbusch

As long as it is perfectly clear that I am expert on nothing, I will be glad to comment. I will try to relate not to the details of Sir Dugald's presentation, which I found clear and informative, but rather to focus on the kinds of thoughts that I, as a sociologist with a somewhat different perspective, have about health care and its relationship to perinatal mortality.

The first point, the notion of the distinction between the obstetrical and environmental causes, does something which physicians are eager to do: that is, to separate the physician and the other health care personnel from the environment.

I am not referring really so much to iatrogenic diseases, but rather to the notion that the patient is confronted with a very confusing world. We may think of prospective patients as everybody, that everyone has all sorts of symptoms, and that one of the very real problems in determination of the incidence of disease is the determination of the appropriateness of going to a health practitioner. The communications between physicians and the subject

23

population are crucial in determining the rates of disease, not only the rates as they are determined at the point where a baby dies or does not die, but also at earlier points where there was a greater likelihood of successful intervention.

What we have, and here I am forced to emphasize my own limited experiences in the United States and in Africa, is a situation in which most people don't feel up to par most of the time. Look around the room and just look at those faces. You know that most of us, if we were really forced, could come up with symptoms which would send us quickly to a physician. We have a problem in communicating which symptoms are to be perceived and worthy of producing a call upon some kind of practitioner.

Sometimes, the practitioner puts off the patient, and we develop, not the usual paramedical specialties, but such occupations as witch doctors, chiropractors, and, in general, those who treat the diseases which the general practitioners find themselves incapable of handling.

The first point, then, is that with respect to perinatal disease, one of the great difficulties is the failure to communicate to subject populations which illnesses or malfunctions, particularly in the case of the mother, are most worthy of reporting to the physician in order to get medical care.

A second point was alluded to by Sir Dugald. I am referring to the importance of longitudinal approaches. Most physicians think they are doing pretty well most of the time, judging by my discussions with people practicing here at Stanford. We have studies, though, for example, at Cornell in New York, that show that when students are assigned to particular patients and follow them up, the students are shocked to discover that all those people who never came back were, in fact, not cured, but rather just went to another kind of practitioner, or just said, "The hell with it," or in many cases did not follow the physician's advice and got well anyway.

The importance of the longitudinal approach is that we may learn about the adequacy of the medical care which we provide, rather than trying to work with broad populations, lacking data on the impact of the physician's intervention.

My third point is rather frightening. And again, Sir Dugald alluded to it as he pointed to the importance of the depression and the results 20, 30, and more years later. We have the problem of following generations with the possibility that significant events now occurring within the lives of individuals are going to have a tremendous impact upon their behavior much later.

This is complicated by the mobility of the American population, which is a real problem for research. We have, for example, the possibility that drug usage today is going to have tremendous implications for obstetrics and pediatrics in the very distant future. We simply do not know, especially as drug usage gets down to the elementary schools, what the implications of this usage will be. It is certainly going to take an unusual physician to examine the particular symptoms that he observes in his practice or researches on disease incidence and then try to say what could have happened to that cohort at an earlier period in time. It really makes a most difficult area for clinical investigation.

Now, related to this is a point to which Dr. Kaiser also alluded. It is the problem of communication between the physician and the patient, particularly with respect to certain kinds of social similarities. We have research on children which shows that they tend to model their behavior or imitate those who are like them in age, in sex, social class, or even sharing similar physical disability.

In the practice of medicine and in the organization of medical care, we often find a tremendous discrepancy between the social characteristics of those who are practitioners and those who are their patients. It is my belief that one of the ways in which paramedical personnel can best be used is to recognize the great social barriers between the usual practitioner and the patient, and to use paramedical personnel so as to provide a way of getting some degree of similarity between those who give advice or inquire about symptoms. This gives a sense of warmth and concern based on greater similarity between those persons and those whom they are treating. It seems to me that one way we can reorganize medical care is to change the communication matrix and, thereby, increase the likelihood of women with particular kinds of problems going to physicians at an earlier stage, thus influencing later perinatal mortality. This attempt will use paramedical personnel so that those who are treating the patient are more like the patient.

Sociologists are often asked by physicians to tell them about changes in values, about how society is shifting and how these shifts relate to the practice of medicine. Let us consider the importance, for example, of the age of the mother. I just want to assure you, on the basis of all the research that I know, that sociologists, like other social scientists, are completely unable to tell you anything worthwhile about what I would call collective dispositions. For example, we have fashions in women. Part of the relative decline since the 1930's in the proportion of women, compared to men, going on to higher education at the A.B., M.A. and Ph.D. levels is a product not only of discrimination but of changing fashions regarding the female role. We are about to see a remarkable change in what happens to women in their career plans and in the age of the mothers at first birth. We simply do not know when or whether they will have second, third, or fourth births.

These changing values are going to have great impact upon perinatal mortality and on the incidence of particular diseases. These value changes are swift, and, to a large extent, they are unexplained. We simply don't understand how value shifts relate to the population.

I would like to close with one final topic, the organization of medical care. It is an important part of a sociological approach to perinatal mortality.

Put very briefly, we can have two kinds of ways of organizing complexities. One is the professional, the person who has internalized certain standards, values, and techniques. He can do what is necessary. The other is the bureaucratic or hierarchical situation in which the tasks are assigned to different persons. They are allocated goals. Each person is evaluated on his performance and, on the basis of these evaluations, differential rewards are distributed. Thereby each person is pressured to contribute to the total operation.

In medical care today we have most professionals practicing in bureaucracies. This produces a revolution in the physician's relationship to the patient and his colleagues. We are moving to a world in which professionals are no longer independent practitioners and must relate to each other.

The evaluation process in a mixed professional bureaucracy is an extremely difficult one. One study at a medical center not too far from here showed, for example, that the physicians believed that they were very important evaluators to the nurses, that the nurses really cared greatly about the physicians' opinion of the nurses' work. In reality, such was the feeling of the nurses about the work load that the physicians placed upon them and the nurse's perception of the lack of competence of physicians to determine appropriate timing for the work, that about half of the nurses did not name a single physician as important to them in any way in the evaluation of their work.

Another study played the game the other way. A colleague, Elliot Freidson, found that the notion of clinical self-control is also unrealistic. In his studies of group practice, most of the physicians were too busy caring for patients to look at each other's performance.

I end with these comments because I believe, as did our keynote speaker last night, that we are moving toward much more group practice; that we are trying to provide a higher level of medical care for all, regardless of ability to pay; and that we should realize at this time that we need research. We should study not just patients, not just physicians, but the interaction of patients and physicians, the ways in which they communicate one with another, and the environment in which the physicians are practicing. These kinds of social environments are just as crucial and just as important as the other environments upon which Sir Dugald so aptly commented.

Sociological Considerations of Maternal and Infant Capabilities

General Discussion

Discussion following Dr. Baird's and Dr. Dornbusch's papers was started by Dr. Kaiser who raised the question, "Is an individual who reproduces during her middle and late teens really subject to more difficulty during her pregnancy and a higher perinatal mortality, as Sir Dugald's statistics would indicate?" Both Dr. Baird's and Dr. Dornbusch's answers revolved around the fact that statistics may not give the entire answer. The social class of the teenage pregnant patient is usually one of the lower social classes. This may be responsible for the higher perinatal mortality. It was then pointed out that it is very difficult to separate all the factors operating in the teenage pregnancy and indeed difficult to separate the various factors operating within social classes. Dr. Hellman mentioned that some excellent results in perinatal mortality have been obtained in teenage pregnancy from lower social classes, i.e., Sarrel study at Yale.

The discussion then began to revolve around ways one could analyze the factors affecting perinatal mortality, both Dr. Kass and Dr. Minkowski stressing the benefits occurring from the use of multifactorial analysis. Various factors,

27

such as maternal complications (i.e., diabetes, toxemia, etc.), social class, parity, and nutrition, were discussed with the general consensus that the data available, in many instances, were poor, and frequently when data were available, conflicting results were reported in different studies. For example, correlating maternal nutrition (weight gain) and fetal weight or fetal outcome, in one study the correlation is poor and in another it is good. A strong point was made that even when one uses a multivariant analysis, correlation does not mean causation. Discussion of how to do such a study returned to multifactorial analysis plus using a homogenous, well followed, easily accessible population. It was concluded that though the problems in such studies are legion, the information is necessary.

Infection

Introduction

James Metcalfe

The concern, this afternoon, is to identify maternal characteristics associated with perinatal morbidity and mortality. As a physician for adults, I have two concerns besides the immediate emphasis of this conference. The first is that pregnancy, considered as a complicated series of biological events, is a time when testing for the health of the individual is particularly important. Successful pregnancy, whether in animals or in humans, is an index of health.

The second bias is that some questions can be more appropriately answered in animal models than in humans. I believe that this proposition is relevant, particularly in view of the objections raised concerning whether this is the correct time, or ethical, political, or economic place, to respond to these questions by utilizing humans for the investigation.

Edward Kass will review the evidence for an association between maternal infection and prematurity. Then Charles Alford will expand upon the role of viruses in perinatal health.

Infection and Maternal and Infant Capabilities

Edward Kass

The importance of the effect of nutrition on pregnancy and the conceptus is not clear. We reviewed some of the critical problems of assessing the significance of sociologic and nutritional data. The data as we know them do not indicate, in most populations in the Western world, a major effect of nutrition on the outcome of pregnancy. The data also do not reflect a high rate of sufficient nutritional deficiency to account for the adverse effects of socioeconomic class on the outcome of pregnancy. Carefully conducted studies are required to examine this problem, but even with adequate nutrition the basic problem of why the poor have more low birth weight deliveries still remains unanswered. For alternative hypotheses to poor nutrition as related to low birth weight, we must resort to clinical observation.

The clinical observation that relates infection to the outcome of pregnancy about which there is no disagreement are the observations made before the advent of specific antimicrobial therapy; when a pregnant woman developed clinically apparent infection, the outcome of the pregnancy tended to be adversely affected.[8,10]

It is unquestionable that increased perinatal mortality and increased prematurity are a consequence of symptomatic infection. Since the most common symptomatic infection of pregnancy is pyelonephritis, one can conclude that symptomatic pyelonephritis causes adverse effects on the outcome of pregnancy.

The mechanisms by which any of these effects occur are unknown. Whatever those mechanisms are, it is conceivable that they could be mimicked by infections that produce less symptomatic responses in a patient. This question, simple enough in concept, has aroused uncommon emotion, probably because in the asking one becomes involved in broad epidemiological approaches that require a degree of expertise that is often not understood.

Asymptomatic infections of the urinary tract, the commonest infection of pregnancy, will be used as our model. The first observations published showed that asymptomatic bacteriuria occurred in 4 to 7 percent of pregnant women. If these pregnant women were given a placebo, there was about a 20 percent risk of their developing symptomatic pyelonephritis during the pregnancy. About 15 percent more would develop symptomatic pyelonephritis during the first postpartum year. If the bacteria were eliminated from the urinary tracts of these individuals, the risk of developing symptomatic disease decreased to exceedingly low levels (Table I and II).

This simple observation initially stimulated considerable controversy. The observations have been reproduced in so many countries and in so many populations, indicating that these results were true, although the rate of bacteriuria is not constant for different populations. There are indications of a socioeconomic gradient in the rate of bacteriuria for reasons not at all clear.

TABLE I. Prematurity Rates in Relation to Symptoms

Group	No. Deliveries	No. Prematures	% Prematurity
Symptomatic Patients			
Random Sample	7	2	28.6
Placebo	26	4	15.4
Misc. Bact.	21	4	19.1
Presumptive Bact.	24	5	20.8
Asymptomatic Patients			
Random Sample	478	65	13.3
Treated & Cleared	75	6	8.0
Treated & Not Cleared	18	1	5.6
Placebo Bact.	72	17	23.6
Misc. Bact.	19	5	26.3
Presumptive Bact.	110	18	16.4

Reprinted, by permission, from Savage, W. E., Hajj, S. N. and Kass, E. H.: "Demographic and prognostic characteristics of bacteriuria in pregnancy." Medicine 46 (5) 399, 1967. (Courtesy of The Williams and Wilkins Co.).

TABLE II. Prematurity Rates in Bacteriuric and Treated Patients

Group	Total No. Deliveries	Twin Deliveries	Total Prematures		Prematures Excl. Twins	
			No.	%	No.	%
1. Random Sample	496	6	67	13.5	57	11.5
2. Treated Bact.	93	0	7	7.5	7	7.5
3. Placebo Bact.	98	3	21	21.4	15	15.3
a. Treated (Symptomatic)	26	0	4	15.4	4	15.4
b. Untreated	72	3	17	23.6	11	15.3
4. Misc. Bact.	40	2	9	22.5	5	12.5
5. Presumptive Bact.	134	1	23	17.2	21	15.7

Reprinted, by permission, from Savage, W. E., Hajj, S. N. and Kass, E. H.: "Demographic and prognostic characteristics of bacteriuria in pregnancy." Medicine 46 (5) 397, 1967. (Courtesy of The Williams and Wilkins Co.).

Higher socioeconomic groups seem to have lower rates of bacteriuria than do lower socioeconomic groups. Our data relate only to the lowest socioeconomic groups served by the Boston City Hospital. Data obtained from other social groups are needed.

The additional observation was made that those women whose bacteriuria was associated with later development of symptomatic pyelonephritis had a higher rate of prematurity than those women who showed no symptoms.

From this information it follows that symptomatic pyelonephritis of pregnancy can be prevented by eliminating bacteriuria. Then, the excess rate of prematurity associated with symptomatic disease would also be prevented. This conclusion must be valid unless those women who are likely to develop symptomatic disease and to have premature delivery have some underlying condition predisposing to both problems. This question remains incompletely resolved, since the prompt treatment of symptomatic pyelonephritis does not completely eliminate the excessive risk of prematurity. Unfortunately, the confirmations of these observations were cluttered by poorly executed studies, which have been adequately reviewed elsewhere. As more careful studies emerged, identification of the woman with bacteriuria became more clearly understood and a number of large-scale studies were published which clarified the situation.

For example, the data of Condie et al. in London showed that when bacteriuria was identified at the Edgware Hospital, the rate of prematurity in nonbacteriuric women was less than in women with bacteriuria.[3] Similar data have now been obtained in Germany, Sweden, Denmark, several parts of the United States, South America, and other areas. There is no question but that the rate of prematurity is about two times greater when bacteriuria is present than when it is absent.

Since the overwhelming majority of women with bacteriuria are spared premature delivery, it becomes important to identify high risk people within the already delimited high risk group of women with bacteriuria.

A beginning to this separation of high risk individuals is based on the observation that if treatment of the pregnant woman is given on a short-term basis, and the patients followed to see who has not responded or who has suffered a recurrence, those who did not respond well to treatment seem to have most of the premature deliveries (Table III).

TABLE III. Prematurity, Mean Birth Weight, Fetal Mortality and Bacteriuria

	Bacteriurics	Controls
Total Cases	180	180
Premature babies		
(2,500 g or less at birth)	23 (12.8%)	9 (5%)
Mean birth weight	6 lbs, 13.5 ozs	7 lbs, 3.3 ozs
Fetal mortality		
Stillbirths	2	0
Neonatal deaths	4	1
Abortions	3	1

Adapted, by permission, from O'Grady, F. and Brumfitt, W. (Eds.): *Urinary Tract Infection.* London, Oxford Univ. Press, 1968, pp. 156, 157.

Thus, in the data from Brumfitt's laboratory, Group I represents those patients whose bacteriuria clears and the urine remains clear for the remainder of pregnancy; these patients are easy to treat. Group II represents those whose bacteriuria either fails to clear or whose bacteriuria returns promptly after two weeks of treatment. Group IIA are the cases in whom bacteriuria returned, and IIB are the ones whose bacteriuria never cleared. In general, those patients in whom treatment for bacteriuria is difficult are the ones who have premature infants. This same group of patients also have an excessive rate of stillbirth and neonatal death. Similar data have been obtained in our laboratory by Elder *et al.* (Table IV).

Another interesting finding, which at the moment cannot be evaluated because of insufficient information, is that the rate of congenital anomalies is greater in children born to women with bacteriuria. Kincaid-Smith and Bullen, in Australia, have reported a similar trend in patients with bacteriuria. It is not determined whether these results are related to maternal anomalies of the urinary tract in patients with bacteriuria so that these women may have offspring who reflect the increased rate of maternal anomalies, or whether this finding indicates the presence of a chronic and unsuspected infection which may affect the outcome of the development of the fetus. In the rat, it is possible to produce congenital anomalies by administering bacterial endotoxin at the correct point in pregnancy.

TABLE IV. Outcome of Pregnancy in Tetracycline-Treated
Bacteriuric Patients

		Cleared and Remained Clear	Cleared then Recurred	Did not Clear
Gestation	mean	38.4	39.	38.
Length	S.D.	2.72	3.3	2.8
(weeks)	n	83	15	9
Birth	mean	109.5	106.	107.
Weight	S.D.	17.3	20.8	25.6
(ounces)	n	83	15	9
Low birth	n	10	4	3
Weight	%	10.1	21.	20.

Adapted, by permission, from Elder, H. A., Santamarina, B. A. G., Smith, S. and Kass, E. H.: "The natural history of asymptomatic bacteriuria during pregnancy: the effect of tetracycline on the clinical course and the outcome of pregnancy." Amer. J. Obstet. Gynec. 111: 441-462, 1971. (Courtesy of The C. V. Mosby Company).

The relation between bacteriuria and later pyelonephritis has been repeatedly demonstrated in many different types of studies throughout the world. There is almost no pyelonephritis of pregnancy in those women who do not have bacteriuria at the first prenatal screening. There are a small number of women who demonstrate bacteriuria as the pregnancy progresses and some of these may become symptomatic.

There are a number of other relationships between bacteriuria and the outcome of pregnancy. Data from the West Indies by Stuart and his associates show that women with bacteriuria had twice the rate of prematurity as women without bacteriuria; the effects were most striking in those women who were hypertensive and who also demonstrated bacteriuria. Bacteriuria seems to interact with other conditions to lead to an excess rate of prematurity.[11]

Similarly, Pometta et al. studied pregnant diabetic women in the Joslin Clinic. If such women had retinopathy and bacteriuria, they lost 50 percent of their babies. If they had retinopathy without bacteriuria, they lost only 15 percent of their babies.[9]

Another argument indicating the role of bacteriuria on the outcome of pregnancy is a finding mentioned earlier. The correlation between birth weight and maternal weight in normal nonbacteriuric women is approximately .25. If bacteriuria had an independent effect on the weight of the child, then one would expect a different correlation coefficient in women with bacteriuria and their infants. In fact, the correlation coefficient is not significantly different from zero, but is significantly (p < .01) different from the coefficient usually obtained from normal infants and women.

How can the woman with bacteriuria who is particularly likely to deliver a small infant be detected? Women who are difficult to treat seem more likely to have an abnormal outcome. Also the hemagglutinin titer against the organism found in the urine was predictive of who was going to be sick many weeks later. The women who had the highest hemagglutinin titers were the most likely to become sick later possibly associated with substantial invasion of the tissues. Similarly, it is well known that women with bacteriuria often have a concentrating defect and cannot concentrate above 700-800 mOsm. If one looks for urinary concentration defects, then the poorer the capacity to concentrate the urine, the greater is the risk of development of symptomatic pyelonephritis of pregnancy. Concentrating ability and elevated antibody both seem to indicate some type of renal infection and predict those patients who are likely to become symptomatic.

If the patients were divided on the basis of their capacity to concentrate their urine and then divided on the basis of whether they responded to two weeks of sulfonamide with success or failure—that is, whether or not they cleared the bacteriuria for the rest of pregnancy, those who concentrated well experienced a 76 percent success rate; whereas, those who concentrated poorly had a 33 percent success rate. The mean difference in maximal osmolality in the two groups was similar; those who had a high failure rate having significantly poorer mean concentration than those with successful treatment. So those women who enter pregnancy with a concentration defect are (a) more difficult to treat successfully, and (b) more likely to become acutely symptomatic. One would infer that they are the women who are particularly likely to deliver small infants.

By discriminant analysis, one can compare hemagglutinin titer with osmolality. These measurements are closely correlated, but osmolality provides all the data, and the antibody titer adds no predictive information.

In summary, among women with bacteriuria we can delimit those who are particularly premature-prone by finding those who do not respond optimally to a short course of therapy. These in turn seem to be the ones who have evidence of renal invasion by bacteria as manifested by their greater rate of diminished concentrating ability and by higher antibody titers.

Dr. Zinner and I have been concerned with what happens to these people many years later. We have a follow-up 10 to 12 years after the first study, which we did in 1956-60. Roughly a quarter of those who had bacteriuria the first time had bacteriuria at follow-up. These were all treated. Of the 98 who did not have bacteriuria in the 1967-69 follow-up, and then were restudied in 1970, another 22 percent developed bacteriuria. Thus, the turnover is about 25 percent per annum. This is a high risk group. In the women who initially did not have bacteriuria, only 5 percent had bacteriuria on follow-up. That is exactly what would be expected. This suggests that bacteriuria in pregnancy delineates a group of patients who are destined to have excessive rates of bacteriuria later in life.

Kunin has followed this problem carefully in school children and finds rates of infection and of turnover that are consistent with the data in adults.[7] What is important, is how many of these have associated renal disease. We could not get all the women in for pyelography, but of the ones who had bacteriuria in the first follow-up (there were 51) we obtained pyelographic studies in 29. We then brought in random nonbacteriuric control women seen in 1956-1959. There were 8 women with bacteriuria who were considered by two radiologists (reading blindly) as having chronic pyelonephritis. Two of these had papillary necrosis; neither of them took analgesics or were diabetic. We presume this was related to the infection.

From calculations, we conclude that 8 to 10 percent of all women with bacteriuria in pregnancy will at a follow-up 10 or 12 years later have pyelographic changes that are diagnostic of chronic pyelonephritis. Because we did not do pyelographic studies in the original population, we cannot tell how many had pyelonephritis at the index pregnancy.

Compared with rates found in England in two separate studies, our rate is higher. We are uncertain whether it is because we followed the patients longer or because our criteria were different. This is a difficult problem to resolve.

Screening for bacteriuria is cheap and easy. The cheapest and easiest test is presently the slide test in which a little puddle of nutrient agar is put on one side of a glass slide and inhibitory agar on the other. The slide is dipped into the urine and put back in the vial. The entire process takes about two seconds. From the density of colonies, one gets an accurate colony count. Obviously, paramedical personnel will be able to perform the entire procedure at relatively low cost.

One must remember that the most important variable in searching for bacteriuria is how the patient is cleansed. The optimal way to cleanse the patient for urine culture is to use ordinary liquid soap as a vigorous wash applied four separate times, each with a large gauze sponge. We find also that in general it is better that the patient be carefully instructed to wash herself.

There are reliable methods for determining whether the contamination rate is adequately low or whether it is excessive. These methods have been published for many years and are slowly beginning to be understood as an application of concepts of study of error in any technique. It is sufficient to say that until a laboratory studies the error in its own method, the data on bacteriuria from the laboratory must be considered suspect.

Finally, a curious observation was made in 1959 that ultimately led us to new directions. We were interested, at that time, in the best way to treat bacteriuria. Dr. Elder studied a series of people using tetracycline. (This was before the tooth staining problem had been recognized.) Since tetracycline seems to improve the body weight of livestock, it was appropriate to have a control group of women who did not have bacteriuria to see if tetracycline affected the outcome of pregnancy through an effect on body weight of the mother.

To our surprise, tetracycline in a double-blinded placebo study in women who did not have bacteriuria lowered the rate of low birth weight significantly and had no effect on maternal weight. This unexpected information required further study. Hence, a double-blinded study of 1200 consecutive women who had no bacteriuria was constructed. By 1960, we reproduced the earlier findings.

Since the dental staining problem was now beginning to be appreciated, we felt it essential to perform follow-up studies of the children before publishing the data. We have completed a six-year follow-up of the children. The second teeth are not stained, and there is no effect on growth and development, as determined by two dentists and two pediatricians. Each examined the children without knowing the treatment history of the mothers. Comparisons between the placebo and drug groups showed no significant demographic differences in the mothers to account for the differences in birth weight of their offspring.

The findings now led to the question: Are there unrecognized asymptomatic infections in the pregnant woman that might be due to microorganisms other than the known ones? A detailed study of the microbial flora of the female genital tract suggested that genital mycoplasmas might qualify. Methods were set up to isolate T-strain mycoplasmas and *M. hominis* as the two mycoplasmas most commonly found in the genital tract. Both of these species are susceptible to tetracycline, and further study confirmed that T-strains are relatively resistant to lincomycins and susceptible to erythromycin, whereas *M. hominis* is relatively susceptible to the lincomycins and relatively resistant to erythromycin. Thus the drugs can be incorporated into the media and used to isolate each species selectively.

A large consecutive series of cervical and vaginal cultures showed that in our pregnant population about 80 percent had mycoplasmas in the genital tract. Specifically, in 568 consecutive pregnant women, the rate of isolation of one or another of the mycoplasmas was 84 percent from cervix plus urine, 78 percent in cervix and 73 percent in urine alone. It might be added that mycoplasmas are highly sensitive to soap, so the patient must be washed with water or saline.

The women, cultured at the first prenatal visit, were followed to term. In the women who had no mycoplasma, the mean birth weight was not different from the mean birth weight of those who had *M. hominis* alone, but was substantially different from the birth weight of the patients who had T-strains alone. There is a striking effect in those who have H plus T.[2]

Dr. Jerome Klein was simultaneously studying cultures from the noses and throats of newborn infants. If the newborn infant was small, the rate of isolation of mycoplasmas was substantially higher than if the newborn infant was larger.

What about the genital mycoplasmas? We, along with Foy *et al.* in Seattle, have observed the same phenomenon, i.e., that mycoplasmas are more commonly found in blacks than in whites.[5] From this, we would like to infer a socioeconomic relationship, but the data to prove this are by no means established. However, the mean birth weights of the children are substantially different in blacks than in whites, in the presence of T-strains in the mother. There is a 9-ounce difference in birth weight according to whether the children were born to T-strain positive or negative black mothers. No difference was found in relation to whether *M. hominis* was present, even though blacks are much more likely than whites to harbor *M. hominis* (Table V).

TABLE V. Presence of Genital Mycoplasmas[a] at First Prenatal Visit in Relation to Gestational Length and Birth Weight[b]

		Birth Weight* (oz)		Gestational Length (wks)[†]		t Tests of Birth Weight	
Group	N	Mean	S.D.	Mean	S.D.	Group	p
1. Negative	78	114.6	17.9	39.3	2.3	1 vs 2	.062
2. Positive for *M. hominis* only	22	122.6	17.2	39.9	2.2	1 vs 3	.259
3. Positive for T-strains only	177	111.4	21.4	39.3	3.0	1 vs 4	.006
4. Positive for *M. hominis* and T-strains	207	107.3	20.5	39.0	3.0	2 vs 3	.019
						2 vs 4	.002
Total	434	110.7	20.6	39.2	2.9	3 vs 4	<.057
						1,2 vs 3,4	.003
*$F = 5.441$, $p < .002$		[†]$F = .723$, $p = .539$				1,3 vs 2,4	<.054

[a]Cultures taken from cervix and urine: isolates from either source considered positive.

[b]Birth weights and gestational lengths include multiple births, births by Caesarean section, and weights of abortuses and stillbirths.

Adapted, by permission, from Braun, P., Yhu-Hsiung, L., Klein, J. O., Marcy, S. M., Klein, T. A., Charles, D., Levy, P. and Kass, E. H.: "Birth weight and genital mycoplasmas in pregnancy." New Eng. J. Med. 284 (4) 168, 1971. (Courtesy Massachusetts Medical Society).

The numbers of patients with pure *M. hominis* were very small, but broken down on a white-black basis, this reflects almost completely the difference in racial distribution. Whites have bigger babies than blacks, and were more likely than blacks to have a pure culture of *M. hominis*. In the large series, as in Dr. Klein's earlier series, the smaller the baby, the higher the rate of colonization with T-strains.

On the other hand, in whites, the presence or absence of T-strain is associated with a 5-ounce difference in birth weight, but yielded an r of .08. If this trend were to continue for twice the size of the population, it would be significant. Yet this is only an inference. Overall, T-strains in the mother have a highly significant relation to low birth weight ($p < .002$).

The only significant correlate with isolation of mycoplasmas has been with mild fever in the postpartum period. Those who carry T-strains have more maternal fever than those who do not. There are now several case reports in which *M. hominis* has been isolated from the blood of patients with postpartum fevers. There are some data on Cesarean sections to indicate that mycoplasmas are uncommon in babies delivered by section. To summarize, it appears a new area for investigation has evolved, i.e., the role of mycoplasma in abnormal outcomes of pregnancy. I must once again stress that data at present represent only high association and not proof that these are causative.

An important problem now must be considered. When is it justified to do a therapeutic trial with antimicrobial agents under conditions of this sort in an asymptomatic woman? It is my conviction that many of the abnormalities of pregnancy are environmental in origin. It seems reasonable that we must expect that a certain number of environmental agents will be infectious. Other types of external agents must also be expected to play a role.

It is reasonable to anticipate that one of the ways of coping with these external agents is with the appropriate use of drugs. The problem arises in using drugs for highly important and justifiable purposes under circumstances in which it is considered unjustified to do so.

Carefully thought out and carefully controlled studies, carefully designed and carefully supervised, are necessary in limited numbers as a way of determining the usefulness of certain drugs in reducing abnormalities of pregnancy. The drugs would have to be chosen very carefully, but given data such as the T-strain data, there is no real alternative to attempting a therapeutic trial. Yet the interdictions are strong and there is a serious problem about how we ought to progress in lowering the rate of prematurity under these circumstances.

I do not mean to slight other possible infectious agents, because I believe they must be numerous. I have presented the two in which the data are the strongest. Data on cytomegalovirus will be presented with respect to congenital anomalies. These data are sufficiently suggestive to require more research. A case can be made for looking into Herpes hominis II, and perhaps into toxoplasma.

There are unexplored possibilities for accounting for excess prematurity in certain high risk groups. If one looks at socioeconomically deprived populations, nutrition is not the only variable that separates them from the more affluent. Infection is one of the most powerful factors that separates the two. If we look at only one of these differentiating factors, we may be missing important information.

BIBLIOGRAPHY

1. Abramowicz, M., Kass, E. H., "Pathogenesis and Prognosis of Prematurity," New Eng. J. Med. 275: 878-885, 938-953, 1001-1007, 1053-1059 (1966).

2. Braun, P., Lee, Y. H., Klein, J.O., Marcy, S.M., Klein, T.A., Charles, D., Levy, P., Kass, E.H., "Birth Weight and Genital Mycoplasmas in Pregnancy," New Eng. J. Med. 284: 167-171 (1971).

3. Condie, A.P., Williams, J.D., Reeves, D.S., Brumfitt, W., "Complications of Bacteriuria in Pregnancy," *Urinary Tract Infection,* ed. by F. O'Grady and W. Brumfitt, London, Oxford University Press, 148-159 (1968).

4. Elder, H.A., Kass, E.H., "Excess Prematurity in Tetracycline-Treated Bacteriuric Patients Whose Infection Persisted or Returned," *Antimicrobial Agents and Chemo-therapy—1967,* ed. by G.L. Hobby, Ann Arbor, American Society for Microbiology 101-109 (1968).

5. Foy, H.M., Kenny, G.E., Wentworth, B.B., *et al.,* "Isolation of *Mycoplasma hominis,* T-strains, and Cytomegalovirus from the Cervix of Pregnant Women," Am. J. Obstet. Gynec. 106: 635-643 (1970).

6. Kincaid-Smith, P., "Bacteriuria in Pregnancy," *Progress in Pyelonephritis,* ed. by E.H. Kass, Philadelphia, F.A. Davis Co., 11-26 (1965).

7. Kunin, C.M., "Epidemiology of Bacteriuria and Its Relation to Pyelonephritis," J. Infect. Dis. 120: 1-9 (1969).

8. Norden, C.W., Kass, E.H., "Bacteriuria of Pregnancy—A Critical Appraisal," Ann. Rev. Med. 19: 431-470 (1968).

9. Pometta, D., Rees, S.B., Younger, D., Kass, E.H., "Asymptomatic Bacteriuria in Diabetes," New Eng. J. Med. 276: 1118-1121 (1967).

10. Savage, W.D., Hajj, S.N., Kass, E.H., "Demographic and Prognostic Characteristics of Bacteriuria in Pregnancy," Medicine 46: 385-407 (1967).

11. Stuart, K.L., Cummins, M.B., Chin, W.A., "Bacteriuria, Pre-ecalmptic Toxemia, and Prematurity, *Progress in Pyelonephritis,* ed. by E.H. Kass, Philadelphia, F.A. Davis Co., 45-49 (1965).

Infection and Maternal
and Infant Capabilities

Discussion

Charles A. Alford

Dr. Kass has just mentioned the subtlety with which common infectious agents, such as the mycoplasma in the cervix and bacteria in the urinary tract, may in some unknown way be associated with adverse effects on the developing human fetus without producing clinical evidence of systemic disease in the mother or in the newborn which is normally equated with tissue invasion. Thus, the subject of the effect of the low grade, chronic, and subclinical infections as environmental factors that may interfere with normal development in the human has been introduced.

In the past, much attention has been given to understanding the pathogenesis, public health control, chemotherapy and prophylaxis of the severe, acute, self-limiting infections of man. This has resulted in the elimination of many of the epidemic scourges in the developing countries of our time, though similar control has not been achieved, to date, in most of the so-called underdeveloped areas where epidemics of infection still represent the major

41

hazard to life and well-being. Along with the correction of many other social and medical evils in the latter areas, the necessity for the establishment of good public health practice directed at the control of common acute infectious disease is obvious and sorely needed before adequate economic structuring can be achieved. One needs only to review the sequence of this development in our own land to appreciate the necessity for mass sanitary controls.

In developing countries, mortality associated with common communicable infectious diseases has been reasonably mastered so that now, control of morbidity rather than mortality, and of the chronic progressive diseases and the more subtle disturbances of development, such as prematurity, have assumed a greater social importance. It has been known for years that infections, such as syphilis, can cause chronic or recurrent disease and need not be limited to acute problems. Thus, even in the new order of priorities, infections must still be given a position of importance, particularly since they represent natural phenomena that are potentially preventable in the future.

Today, I hope to paint a truer picture of the impact of four common infectious agents on disturbance of development both *in utero* and postnatally and to indicate the subtleness of the associated disease states. The four to be discussed are rubella, cytomegalovirus, toxoplasma gondii, and treponema pallidum. All of these have long been known to produce congenital infections which on occasion may be devastating. These agents may frankly invade the product of conception with resultant chronic infection of the fetus that may persist for long periods postnatally. Therefore, it is currently considered that they may all produce continuing low-grade damage long after their original invasion, a view that adds new perspectives to their possible pathogenic potential and suggests that new approaches are needed to assess their true medical significance. In addition, each of these agents is ubiquitous and circulates among the population at a relatively high rate assuring exposure of many susceptible pregnant women. My discussion will be limited to the incidence, clinical spectrum, and host responses of these invasive fetal infections that carry an obvious high risk for permanent developmental damage, especially with respect to CNS and perceptual functions.

Infections have been recognized as one environmental cause of birth defects and developmental abnormalities since the studies on congenital syphilis in the early part of this century, and since Gregg first recognized the teratogenic potential of rubella virus in the early 1940's. Subsequently, a number of clinical epidemiologic surveys were undertaken to assess the true impact of common infections in this regard. The results have been disappointingly variable. This has led to the general belief that, with the exception of rubella, other common infectious agents lack the potential to produce significant amounts of fetal damage. We know now, however, that these studies far underestimated the potential hazards of maternal infections, primarily because they depended upon the presence of clinically evident disease in the mother and baby as their means of assessment.

I would like to emphasize the fact that the great majority of dangerous infections of pregnancy are clinically "silent" in the mother and too subtle to be recognized in the infected newborn. Laboratory monitors are needed to judge the true significance of infections as causes for birth defects and developmental disorders later in life, and to better define the natural histories of these diseases with future therapeutic considerations in mind. To detect the more common subclinical infections, these monitors must be sufficiently practical to be judiciously applied in large-scale screening studies. They should also have the capability to determine the extent of the problem in such a form that they could be available for general use in the segments of our population where need is ultimately defined. The time-honored isolation and serologic procedures currently available for diagnosis of congenital infections pose problems which are far too complicated to permit their use for these purposes. Instead, classic procedures must be confined to small-scale research studies or for diagnosis of less common, severe, suspect cases.

Because they can be more rapidly and easily performed, serologic procedures for detection of antibody are more suitable for screening studies than are the isolation procedures. In the area of congenital infections, however, the use of the routine serologic testing is limited because placental transfer of maternal antibody results in comparable levels of antibody in newborns, whether they are infected or not. For instance, 80 to 90 percent of all neonates are born with rubella antibody as a reflection of previous maternal infection which has not necessarily been recently acquired. Such testing, then, cannot pinpoint the individual newborn who has been at high risk for intrauterine infection. In the past, this has represented the major hurdle in systematic testing to determine the role of infections in the production of fetal damage.

In recent years, it has been demonstrated that the human fetus can muster an immunologic response when appropriately stimulated, and that in many cases infections can provide such a stimulus. Searching for evidence of the fetus's own antibody response seems one way to overcome the problems posed by transfer of maternal antibody. Since the human fetus can form IgM antibody following infection, while the placenta transfers only IgG from the maternal circulation, the detection of IgM antibodies in cord or neonatal sera is a specific marker for recent fetal infection, providing the placental barrier remains intact. These two antibody types can be distinguished by some of the newer immunologic and serologic techniques. Therefore, screening for the presence of fetal IgM antibodies provides a practical laboratory means for re-evaluating the medical significance of congenital infections. In the past three years, we have screened our entire high risk delivery population, some 7,500 newborns, for evidence of fetal antibody production.

Under the program, IgM is measured by immunodiffusion in cord sera obtained from every baby born at our hospital. After exclusion of specimens contaminated by maternal blood, infants who show elevated values are considered to have experienced an increased antigenic load *in utero* and are therefore, subjected to a series of tests to determine the reason for the elevations.

Tests are performed irrespective of the clinical findings in the mother or infant in order to document subclinical disease. Infections are one obvious source of increased intrauterine antigenic stimulation: our studies were consequently designed to detect as many infections as possible in those neonates who were born with increased IgM. Particular emphasis was placed on the diagnosis of the chronic intrauterine infections because of their potential hazard to the developing central nervous system. In addition to classical diagnostic methods, specific IgM fluorescent antibody tests for the rapid detection of congenital syphilis, cytomegalovirus, and toxoplasma infections were evaluated. To assess the practicality of this approach, the tests were applied under controlled conditions in the hospital diagnostic laboratories after initial development of the methods in a research setting.

Some of the results from the use of this approach are shown in Figure 1. By initially screening the population of newborns for increased levels of cord

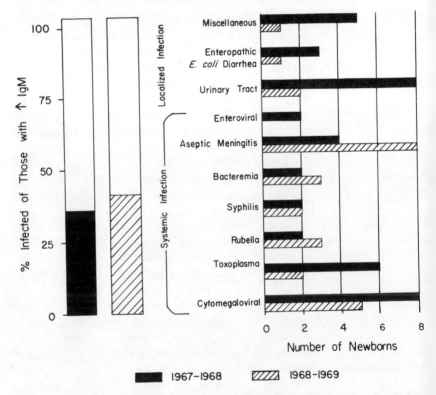

Fig. 1. Infections in infants born with Elevated IgM. Reprinted, by permission, from Alford, C.A.: "Immunologic status of the newborn." Hosp. Pract. 5:(6)92, June 1970. (Courtesy of Hospital Practice.)

IgM, a small group of babies at high risk for infection were defined: this permitted the intensity of studies that were originally performed. Definition of a small high risk group is especially important when initially attempting to define the rate and role of subclinical infections in low socioeconomic populations, such as ours, where many other intrauterine factors, including malnutrition and the like, may adversely influence subsequent development in the same way as infections. Strict control groups must be included if the long term effects of any one of these factors is to be properly assessed. This cannot be adequately done if the study population is too large at the outset.

Only 123 infants with increased IgM levels were found among the 2,916 babies examined in the first year of the study. Infections were detected in 42, or 34 percent, of the infants born with elevated levels of IgM. Diseases identified included 8 cases of cytomegalovirus infection; 6 of toxoplasma infection; 2 of rubella; 2 of syphilis; 2 of bacteremia; 4 of aseptic meningitis, and a group with localized infections. Of the 3,035 sera examined in the second year, there were elevated IgM levels in only 69. In 27, or 39 percent of the neonates born with increased IgM levels, specific infections diagnosed included 5 cases of cytomegalovirus infection; 2 of toxoplasmosis; 3 of rubella; 2 of syphilis; 3 with bacteremia; 8 with aseptic meningitis, and again a few with localized infections.

The infection rate among infants who are born with elevated cord IgM levels was found to be increased 42-fold over those who are born with more normal values. Clearly, the results indicate that infection is one, but not necessarily the only determinant of high IgM values that develop *in utero*. Though it is not a complete epidemiologic tool, screening for elevated cord IgM values can be used as a practical initial step to determine incidence and to better define the nature of intrauterine infections that occur in a given population of newborns. This nonspecific screening technic defines the relative importance of each of these infections; specific methods can then be designed for rapid detection of those that occur at significant rates. For instance, in our studies, cord sera collected from all newborns with congenital syphilis, toxoplasma, rubella, and cytomegalovirus infection contained specific fetal IgM antibodies which were detectable by fluorescent microscopy. Like IgM determinations, these latter tests can be rapidly and economically performed in the hospital diagnostic laboratories. The four chronic congenital infections can, therefore, be diagnosed soon after delivery even in subclinical forms. However, before such testing can be set up in any given service, one must show evidence for need, as the fluorescent antibody tests would have to be used as a battery of screening procedures in order to detect the "silent" infections. This would represent unnecessary expense in a population group where intrauterine infections occurred at an insignificant rate.

The incidence of intrauterine infection in our low socioeconomic predominantly Negro population proved to be surprisingly high: 1 infection per 89 general deliveries. This is particularly striking since the figure must be considered minimal because of the initial screening procedure. A major finding, as noted in Table I, was the high rate of occurrence of the chronic systemic intrauterine infections. This high rate of 1/178 general deliveries has been maintained in each year of the three year study period. If this incidence could be extrapolated to the low socioeconomic segments of our nation or the world at large, it would be truly staggering. More importantly, it emphasizes the continuous potential hazard of even the common infections in certain population groups which are in need of definition. Only chromosomal aberrations vie with infections in this regard and, indeed, infections may themselves contribute to certain forms of chromosomal breakage.

TABLE I.   Incidence of Congenitally-Acquired Infections in 222 Infants
Born with Increased Cord Serum IgM
(2.5 Year Interval)

Type Infection	No	Rate/Infant Born IgM	Rate/General Deliveries[a]
Cytomegaloviral	17	1/13	1/400
Toxoplasmosis	11	1/20	1/682
Rubella	8	1/28	1/938
Syphilis	6	1/37	1/1250
	42	1/5	1/178

[a]Total Deliveries Over 2.5 Year Interval 7500.

Reprinted, by permission, from Alford, C. A.: "Immunoglobulin determinations in the diagnosis of fetal infection." Pediat. Clin. N. Amer. 18: (1), 111, Feb. 1971. (Courtesy of W. B. Saunders, Co.).

As with other populations throughout the world, congenital cytomegalovirus infection proved to be the leading intrauterine infection in our group (Table I). But, surprisingly, congenital toxoplasmosis was the second most common and occurred at a rate in excess of congenital rubella, a disease that has caused considerable alarm in recent years because of its capacity to contribute to developmental difficulty. In our population, congenital syphilis has reached appreciable proportions in keeping with the documented increase in venereal disease among adolescents and young adults in recent years. These data clearly emphasize the need for a re-evaluation of the true impact of intrauterine infections in our people and those in underdeveloped areas.

What is the clinical nature of these infections at delivery? What are their long term effects? Surprisingly, most of the infected newborns were asymptomatic at delivery, irrespective of the infecting agents. Severe disease that produced crippling developmental problems in early life occurred at a rate of approximately 1/1000 general deliveries and was equally associated with each of the four chronic intrauterine infections under discussion. Though this is far less than their actual rate of occurrence (1/178 general deliveries), it is still highly significant when compared to the incidence of such problems as the inborn errors of metabolism, including PKU. We can express these figures in another way: While approximately 10 percent of the chronically infected newborns are delivered with severe damage, these babies still represent a significant input into developmental CNS problems.

What of the more common subclinical infections? As noted in Table II, in spite of the lack of physical findings, more than half of these infants exhibited evidence of central nervous system involvement in the form of elevated spinal fluid protein values and lymphocytosis which persisted for variable but prolonged periods up to five months after delivery. This represents obvious evidence that direct invasion of the developing central nervous system can occur without overt symptoms in the newborn. The four different organisms seem to have differing capabilities in this regard. Toxoplasma and rubella virus produce these changes more often than does cytomegalovirus; they may, therefore, be potentially more hazardous even though they produce intrauterine infection less commonly. The actual medical significance of this type of CNS involvement is poorly defined at present. Long term follow-up will be required to ascertain the total effect on CNS or perceptual development and in producing other signs of illness in later life.

TABLE II. Summary Abnormal CSF Findings in 29 Congenitally Infected Infants Born[a] with Increased IgM

Infections	No. with Abn. CSF/TOT	Abnormal CSF Findings (Range/Mean)		
		Cells (No./cumm)	Protein[b] (mgm/100 cc)	Persistence
Toxoplasmosis	6/6	22-111 (43)	63-1600 (163)[c]	2 wks-5 mo
Rubella	4/8	20-105 (41)	68-245 (106)	1 mo->4 mo
Rubella & Toxoplasmosis	1/1	28-75 (44)	118-245 (164)	>3 mo
Gtomegaloviral	3/10	23-28 (22)	54-108 (75)	5 da-2 wks
Syphilis	1/2	20-140	60-145	21 days
Enteroviral	1/2	119-1311	86-94	14 days
Total	16/29			

[a]Delivered in a 1½ year interval (Aug., 1967-Feb., 1969).

[b]Includes values in all samples with pleocytosis

[c]Calculations exclude values in one infant with inordinately high levels

During the first year of follow-up, a significant proportion of infants showed signs of slowed psychomotor development. Again, this was more common with congenital toxoplasmosis and rubella than with congenital cytomegalovirus infection. Together, these findings suggest that demonstration of inflammatory changes in the spinal fluid at birth are truly a reflection of frank invasion of the substance of the brain *in utero,* and indicate that a large spectrum of CNS damage can be associated with so-called "silent" congenital infections.

Other evidence indicates that adverse effects of these milder congenital infections on fetal development are not necessarily confined to the CNS. For example, the average newborn with subclinical congenital toxoplasmosis had a birth weight 500 g less than the uninfected controls or the average newborn with congenital cytomegalovirus infection. Thus, this disease does seem to cause mild intrauterine growth retardation without other symptoms normally associated with the infection. In addition, the gestational periods of infants with mild congenital toxoplasmosis was shortened by two weeks when compared to controls, suggesting a tendency of this infection to cause premature delivery. There was also an increased incidence of chorioretinitis with otherwise asymptomatic congenital toxoplasmosis. The occurrence of early and, in some cases, sustained hypergammaglobulinemia suggests that immunologic complex disease may also contribute to organ system damage some time later in life. The combination of persistent infection with hypergammaglobulinemia has been demonstrated in all four chronic intrauterine infections. Insufficient time has elapsed to determine the possible effects of immunologic complex disease in infected infants. Clearly, however, our data indicate that the apparent silence of these infections in early life in no way assures that they are harmless.

Some comparative features of congenital cytomegalovirus and toxoplasmosis, which have just been discussed, are graphically depicted in Figure 2. Here it can be seen that severe, debilitating disease occurs at an equal rate with intrauterine infection caused by both of these organisms (rate 1/4500 general deliveries with each). However, significant low-grade brain damage is apparently more common with congenital toxoplasmosis, occurring at a rate of 1/700 general deliveries, while similar low-grade CNS damage with cytomegalovirus occurs at a lower rate of 1/2500 general deliveries. It must be emphasized, though, that as follow-up continues, evidence of low-grade damage may become more apparent in the infants with the latter disease.

One important matter has already become apparent from these studies. We can no longer simply document the presence of infection in the fetus and newborn. We must now predict the severity of the disease in terms of final outcome or any therapeutic regimens designed in the future might become more dangerous than the natural diseases. To do this, it is essential that the causal mechanisms and host response be much better understood than they are currently. It is time that the schizophrenia between the intrauterine and postnatal studies of congenitally acquired infections be ended so that a true

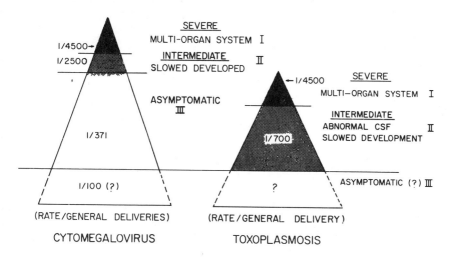

Fig. 2. Comparison of minimal incidence and medical significance of congenital cytomegalovirus and toxoplasma infections.

perinatal approach to understanding these subtle disease states can be achieved. Here, complete cooperation between the obstetrician, neonatalogist, infectious disease expert, pathologist, and pediatrician is mandatory.

In summary, it is now clear, contrary to what was previously believed, that chronic congenital infections are most often silent in both the pregnant mother and her offspring, and that they occur much more commonly than previously thought. A significant number of the infections may in time produce low grade organ damage, especially in the CNS, either because of the pathology incurred *in utero* or, more likely, because of continuing low-grade chronic infection long after delivery. Though recognition in the pregnant mother and early treatment of the fetal infection *in utero* are ideal goals, they may be a long time in coming.

In the meantime, every effort should be made to detect these infections in the newborn and, when possible, to institute therapy to arrest the process. Certainly this approach should contribute to improved performance of infected babies in later life.

BIBLIOGRAPHY

1. Alford, C.A., Foft, J.W., Blankenship, W.J., Cassady, G., Benton, J.W., "Subclinical Central Nervous System Disease of Neonates: A Prospective Study of Infants Born with Increased Levels of IgM," J. Pediat., 75: 1167 (1969).

2. Alford, C.A., "Immunoglobulin Determinations in the Diagnosis of Fetal Infection," Ped. Clin. N. Amer., 18: 99-113 (February, 1971).

3. Courveur, J., Desmonts, G., "Congenital and Maternal Toxoplasmosis, A Review of 300 Congenital Cases," Develop. Med. Child Neurol., 4: 519 (1962).

4. Sever, J.L. (Editor) and Multiple Authors, selected papers on "Immunological Responses to Perinatal Infections," J. Pediat., 75 (1969).

5. Starr, J.G., Bart, R.D., Gold, E., "Inapparent Congenital Cytomegalovirus Infection," New Eng. J. Med., 282: 1075-1078 (1970).

6. Thalhammer, O. (Editor) and Multiple Authors, "Prenatal Infections," International Symposium of Vienna, September 2-3, 1970, Georg Thieme Verlag, Stuttgart (1971).

Infection and Maternal and Infant Capabilities

General Discussion

The discussion that followed the papers of Kass and Alford was opened by Dr. Kass who indicated that the total effect of bacteriuria on infant mortality could not account for more than 10 percent. Hellman added that this would indicate that 5-10 percent of deaths could be prevented, since prematurity accounts for 50-80 percent of neonatal deaths. Kass indicated further that there was a possible relationship of poverty to prematurity and that may be correlated with occurrence of infection. Behrman questioned the spread of the infection from mother to fetus, and Kass said there was no real evidence for this possibility. The fetal membranes were cultured and showed no infectious agent. He thought that in order to follow the problem more realistically, it would be advisable to use immunological tests.

Barnett queried the relationship of gestational age to mortality and rate of infection. The general reply was that gestational age was a very inaccurate figure to compile and that weight of the infant was considerably more accurate. Silverman indicated that he thought that gestational age vs. infant weight was a

51

very important distinction. Barnett thought that the determination of gestational age could be made more accurate by using a variety of new methods, for example, amniocentesis. Greulich pointed out another aspect which was that low weight was a characteristic of the black infant population, but that, in general, they were much more mature. Kass insisted that weight is an objective datum. He agreed that there were racial differences, but that if a large enough group were taken, many of these differences could be ruled out. Behrman emphasized that there were possibilities at present, and certainly more in the future, for determination of gestational age. Kass added to this discussion that the small-for-dates infant may not be the critical factor. Neither may bacteriuria or erythroblastosis be critical factors. He said that the small baby is the end result of a number of phenomena. Kaiser felt that the weight of the baby is associated with mortality. In other words, the smaller the infant the greater the chance for mortality. He felt that the term "prematurity" was vague and almost undefinable except in terms of weight. In fact, the physiological and biochemical aspects of the small-for-dates infant was more important than whether it was defined by weight as premature.

Rossi was impressed by the prevalence of cytomegalovirus. Alford and Kass both pointed out the paucity of data indicating association of cytomegalovirus with small babies, premature delivery, or retardation. Alford said that there was no proof that there is a relationship between cytomegalovirus and any of these end-results. There are two aspects to the problem. One is evidence of antibody to the cytomegalovirus, and the other is actual presence of the virus. Infection with cytomegalovirus is a complex disease which may become manifest later. Rossi asked when the fetus first starts to produce IgM. Alford said that IgM can be measured in cells of the 10-week-old fetus and in the blood at 16-20 weeks.

Segal summarized this portion of the discussion by saying that the term "prematurity" is really unimportant and was generally in agreement with Kaiser that the term was unclear. Kass again responded by indicating that with a proper epidemiological approach many of the problems regarding the use of weight as a standard can be ruled out.

Minkowski emphasized that certain drugs, particularly tetracyclines, may affect the size of the infant. Sereni said that this effect was well known to occur with tetracyclines, that they did result in a decrease in size, particularly by affecting bone growth. It is highly possible that other drugs could do the same thing. Kass pointed out that the investigations of these problems would constitute a series of very difficult studies.

Alford suggested that there should be a general screening program of pregnant women for the many possible infectious diseases. Since there are now a number of screening programs for a variety of genetic diseases, Rosenberg suggested that there could be a series of cooperative studies which would include surveys for genetic problems as well as various viruses, particularly rubella.

Pollution

Introduction

Sydney Segal

Our focus will change from the general environment to the specific environment of the fetus and the newborn infant. We are aware of various pollutants that are presented to the organism: the biophysical ones such as noise; pollution of the air and water; impurities in some drugs; heavy metals which can be absorbed from our environment; and pollutants in human milk. Sir Dugald talked about an irrational tribal custom which was referred to when his daughter wanted to breast-feed her baby. Breast-feeding is a natural process, at least it was a natural process before we polluted our environment. Now, there are insecticides in breast milk, and there is radioactive strontium in some breast milk. Since we realize that our Food and Drug Agency can control the purity of commercial products and can force industry to remove various pollutants from commercial milk, it may be that we have changed our ecology so effectively that natural breast-feeding may no longer be appropriate. Maybe these changes lead to important research questions.

There have been various recent therapeutic misadventures which affected the environment of the fetus and of the newborn. It is particularly appropriate that this group should be discussing the subject of environmental effects on mother and child.

Pollution and Infant Capabilities

Richard Behrman

My purpose is to present some preliminary data concerning several clinical problems that occur during the perinatal period which may be related to the pollution of air.

First, there are epidemiological, statistical type surveys which have many inherent limitations that have been referred to, for example, the problems of correlation and causation. A number of competent people have been looking at the distribution of air patterns and different pollutants. The second general type of information consists of physiologic or chemical measurements, using people or animals subjected to natural or experimentally polluted environments. In spite of the limitations, both approaches add significant though complex perspectives to the biologic effects of air pollutants.

Incidence of specific diseases and associated mortality have been related to a number of indices of air pollution. It has been projected that with bronchitis, mortality could be reduced by 25 or even 50 percent, depending upon the particular location and deposit index, by reducing the pollution to the lowest level currently prevailing in each of these regions.

These particular studies were corrected for socioeconomic backgrounds and available gross pollution indices. The use of the lowest minimum current level prevailing in the regions is a practical correction factor that has to be used by statisticians, since it is difficult to obtain consistent long periods of zero pollution by the particular agents under investigation.

An association has been found between the mortality and morbidity rates for heart disease in adults and the level of air pollution. The morbidity rates are twice as high in polluted areas as in the clean air areas. Mortality rates may be 10 to 20 percent higher in some patients with myocardial infarctions. There are data to suggest that the ambient level of carbon monoxide may play a significant role in reducing the amount of oxygen delivered to the myocardium.

Epidemiologic information with children is very meager. There have been significant correlations found between air pollution and the prevalence of respiratory disease in school children both in Great Britain and in this country, but great caution is needed in interpreting these figures.

There are also significant correlations between air pollution and death rates for all respiratory diseases as well as the morbidity rates for bronchitis and pneumonia. There has been a very tenuous documentation of increased hospitalization rates for children with respiratory disease living in areas of high pollution.

Although respiratory disease remains the principal cause of death in the neonatal period, there is no significant information available about incidence or mortality of specific respiratory diseases during this period in association with increased levels of particulate matter, nitrogen compounds, sulfates, or carbon monoxide in either hospitals or home environments. Although more information will be needed to decide whether a health problem exists in these situations, the adult data are very suggestive. For example, the incidence and severity of viral infections and pneumonia which are quite high in the ghetto areas during the winter may be governed in part by the ambient levels of one pollutant or a combination of different air pollutants adding to the effects of specific infectious pathogens.

It may be that some of the morbidity associated with infections is related principally to their association at the same time with certain air pollutants. This has been suggested by several investigators.

Other studies have demonstrated significant correlations between increases in particulate matter and sulfate pollution in the air and increases in fetal, neonatal, and infant mortality. Lave and Saskin have used some of these data to project the effects of modest decreases in the levels of selected pollutants on the overall mortality figures. These authors developed computer models from the available epidemiologic data. Although based on a number of questionable assumptions, their work raises some interesting questions for future speculation and study.

The data in Table I, adapted liberally from Lave and Saskin, indicate the projected effects of decreased pollution on mortality. The decreases in percent

TABLE I. Projected Effects of Decreased Pollution on Mortality

	Percent decrease in death rate		
	Fetal	Neonatal	Infant
10% decrease in (particles)	0.9	0.6	0.7
10% decrease in (sulfate)	0.5	0.4	0.3
10% decrease in (poor families)	2.0	?	?

Adapted from L. B. Lave and E. P. Saskin

of death rates for the fetal, neonatal, and infant groups are projected in terms of a 10 percent decrease in particulate matter. Particulate matter generally consists of crude particles within well established standard size ranges, as determined on the basis of filtration techniques. Although such techniques have been used for considerable periods of time for industrial purposes, they have not really been used by biologic scientists. The techniques are quite limited, and there are large variations in the information obtained. For example, particulate matter is measured with a very crude instrument which sucks air onto filter paper, weights of the filter paper are obtained and results from the weight and analysis of the filter paper are reported at the end of a month or six months or a year. The effect of variations in humidity at the time the filter paper is taken out of the machine has not been considered. Computer models are used to determine the distribution of a particular pollutant in the area where the mortality data are collected, and these data are then evaluated for correlations with mortality data. Most of the observations are concerned with gaseous sulfur compounds and particulate matter. If the data are reliable and the assumptions are valid, one can project that there would be significant decreases in these mortality rates related to decreases in sulfate fumes or particulate matter. The last line in Table I indicates the effects of a 10 percent decrease in the number of poor families.

I have no experience with which to evaluate the bias of these kinds of data manipulation. Obviously, there are significant political-social implications. However, I think they are worth examining because they provide some indication of the order of magnitude of the potential problem.

I have spoken with some management people in Chicago from a furnace-making company that makes small home furnaces. They say that to decrease the pollution output on a home furnace by 10 percent would add $300 to $400 more to the cost. These are small companies, and they feel the expense would be financially devastating. These are some of the ramifications of the problem.

One of the main problems with these data is that the populations subjected to high levels of residential and industrial urban pollution are often the same populations that are at the lowest socioeconomic levels in society. These are the same populations that have the highest prematurity rate and fetal death rate. It is difficult to correct for these factors, but they must be controlled if we are going to address ourselves to such questions as a causal relationship between high levels of ambient carbon monoxide breathed by pregnant women throughout gestation who live in these areas and a resultant higher fetal death rate. Certainly, association of cigarette smoking and high mortality suggests air pollution may be relevant. There are no data correlating the level of pollution with so-called intrauterine growth retardation.

An understanding of the physiologic mechanisms involved in the vascular responses of the microcirculation of the placenta to low levels of carbon monoxide and the physiologic mechanisms which may play a role in the diffusion of inert gases may also be relevant to answering such questions. Such physiologic investigations may either obviate the necessity for some of the epidemiologic studies, or may aid in determining the most important pollutants.

The physiologic approach to the health effects of air pollution during the perinatal period has received little attention. However, in adults there have been investigations of the direct untoward effects of air pollutants on pulmonary tissue by their action in inducing abnormalities in ventilation-perfusion ratios and abnormalities in diffusion. These studies suggest some basis for understanding mechanisms which play a role in the way that air pollutants may contribute to increasing mortality and morbidity from bronchitis and emphysema. No data are available for the neonatal infant who also has a high incidence of respiratory disease associated with problems of diffusion, ventilation, and perfusion, for example, hyaline membrane disease.

We have recently undertaken an evaluation of the relationship between a decreased oxygen-carrying capacity of hemoglobin in newborn infants and the level of air pollution. Our interest in this problem was a matter of serendipity. We have moved from Oregon which at that time had been a relatively low pollution area. A technician and a veterinarian surgeon moved with me. We all used our own blood to standardize the gas chromatographic apparatus for measuring oxygen-combining capacities. When we started to set up the laboratory in Chicago, using the blood from the same three people (who had not changed their habits—two were nonsmokers, one was a smoker), we found some discrepancies between the calculated oxygen-carrying capacity of hemoglobin and the results we obtained directly on the gas chromatograph. This problem had not been present in Oregon. It took several months to convince ourselves that we were not dealing with a technical or methodologic problem. We then began to investigate the possibility that there might be a difference in the level of air pollution in the laboratory in Chicago that had not existed in Oregon. The University of Illinois hospital is on the edge of a southwestside Chicago ghetto, very close to a freeway and to areas where cheap crude fuel is used to heat homes and businesses.

Our initial data suggested a relationship between days in which there were high pollution levels and decreases in oxygen-carrying capacity. Figure 1 shows the result of a preliminary study. We studied infants in a nursery for newborns,

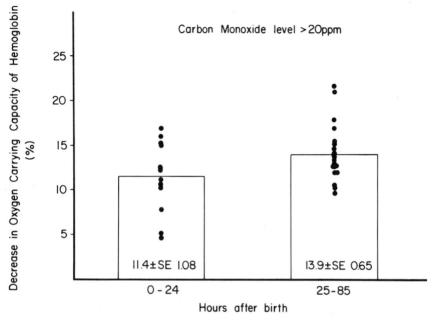

Fig. 1. Relationship between pollution levels and oxygen-carrying capacity of hemoglobin. Reprinted, by permission, from Behrman, R.E., Fisher, D.E., and Paton, T: "Air pollution in nurseries: correlation with a decrease in oxygen-carrying capacity of hemoglobin." J. Pediat. 78:1052, June 1971.(Courtesy of The C.V. Mosby Co.)

on the second floor of the hospital for a possible relation between reduced oxygen-carrying capacity and low pollution days. The level of ambient carbon monoxide was chosen as an index of air pollution, not as a causative agent.[1]

There was a great deal of difficulty obtaining the pollution information. At the time, we had no means of measuring the pollutants ourselves. Because of the vigorous program of the district attorney to control pollution caused by industries, it became very difficult to obtain ambient carbon monoxide levels directly from industry. The information was obtained from Durham rather than directly from the people doing the recording in the city of Chicago.

A number of different pollutants can be recorded. I have referred to particulate matter. Carbon monoxide also can be measured with an infrared spectrophotometer. Sulfates and several nitrogen gaseous compounds are measured with other instruments. The concentration of about 10 compounds in air can be routinely recorded.

In collecting the data on babies, there are certain qualifications. Those infants who, were hemolyzing abnormally had to be excluded from the study. We also eliminated infants born to mothers who smoked during the week before delivery. Carbon monoxide was chosen because the data on this gas were the most accessible and reliable of the various pollutants being measured at that time. Greater than 20 parts per million is called "high" based on experience in the Chicago area. The decrease in oxygen-carrying capacity of hemoglobin is plotted as a percent of the total oxygen-carrying capacity of hemoglobin. This is not a decrease in saturation, but a percent decrease in total oxygen-carrying capacity when the gas chromomatography measured capacity is compared to the capacity calculated from the hemoglobin concentration.

The discrepancy between the two methods we were using in this study, at two standard deviations, is about a 2 percent error. We would expect to find about a 2 percent difference between the oxygen-carrying capacity calculated from the hemoglobin and that determined with a gas chromatograph. There was less than a half percent discrepancy between the gas chromatograph and the Van Slyke method. The gas chromatograph was used because it requires a smaller volume of blood.

We found there was a significant increase in the reduction of oxygen-carrying capacity on days in which the particles of carbon monoxide were greater than 20 parts per million, and that this decrease was greater the longer the baby breathed air in the nursery. Every baby had some indication of air pollution.

This study has a number of limitations. First, the carbon monoxide level was measured at about a mile and a half from the nursery without our supervision. Levels of carbon monoxide were measured continuously in an infrared spectrophotometer. The traffic conditions were different at the place of measurement from the vicinity of the hospital. Also there was the possibility of differences in local use of fuel and proximity to smokestacks. These limitations have led us subsequently to obtain the equipment to measure pollution in our own nursery.

All of these infants were well. There was no physiologic abnormality in any of them. We specifically excluded infants with any type of hemolytic disease on the basis of blood type, reticulocyte counts, smear, or serum bilirubins above 12 g%. We also measured the blood carboxyhemoglobin in this group of infants. This did not make up more than 40 percent of the discrepancy.

This preliminary study raises a number of questions. There is the possibility of a synergistic effect between carbon monoxide and other air pollutants that might account for the decrease in oxygen-carrying capacity. The few remotely related studies deal with adult, not fetal hemoglobin. There is very little known about the effects of low levels of carbon monoxide in combination with sulfates and nitrogenous gases on the fetal oxygen dissociation curve. The classic data had been obtained with high concentrations of carbon monoxide by Haldane on adult blood. Changes in the oxygen affinity of hemoglobins might significantly and detrimentally alter the uptake of oxygen in lungs or its delivery to the tissues in infants with respiratory disease, tissue hypoxia, or both. Such physiologic changes could play a role in increasing the mortality in the neonatal period. Intimately related to these problems and questions are a number of other questions, for example, what are the levels of air pollution of the different pollutants in various areas in the hospital? Only a very few such studies are available.

One of the best studies of this latter question was accomplished a number of years ago at the University of Pennsylvania Hospital before the city grew into close proximity to the hospital. Air was sampled in different parts of the hospital. The level of pollution in the city and hospital was low.

In the late 1950's, because of concern with staphylococcal hospital infections in nurseries, provisions were made in many hospitals to circulate varying proportions of outside air into the nurseries. The filters for this air, as well as for the recirculating hospital air, have no effect on most of the gaseous pollutants. Perhaps such filters now need to be developed. The patterns of air pollution within the hospital need to be mapped in relation to the traffic pattern in the vicinity, the location of the hospital relative to industries and in relation to the equipment and activities going on in a hospital at different times of the day.

For example, there are higher concentrations of carbon monoxide at 11 a.m. than at 3 p.m. in the high risk intensive care unit. At times, the amount of carbon monoxide in internally circulated air is higher than it is in the outside air. At other times, the outside air carbon monoxide is higher than that in the inside air. These changes may be the result of traffic patterns, distribution of heat, and air in the hospital, or the different activities of day and night. We need to have more information about such patterns.

In conclusion, I think one can say that, first, there is suggestive qualitative evidence for an effect of air pollution on health during the perinatal period. Second, that the magnitude and the relative importance of these effects are totally unknown and rarely investigated. Thirdly, both epidemiologic and physiologic studies are needed to focus on problems related to pulmonary disease and tissue oxygenation as related to the quality of air in and outside hospitals.

BIBLIOGRAPHY

1. Behrman, R.E., Fisher, D.E., Paton, J., "Air Pollution in Nurseries: Correlation with a Decrease in Oxygen Carrying Capacity of Hemoglobin," J. Pediat., 78: 1050-1054 (June, 1971).

Pollution and Infant Capabilities

Discussion

Lawrence D. Longo

I would like to consider some biologic implications of carbon monoxide, not only on newborns but on the pregnant mother and the fetus *in utero*.

The carboxyhemoglobin percent saturation is simply the quotient of the carbon monoxide content of the blood and the carbon monoxide capacity multiplied by 100.

$$\text{Carboxyhemoglobin percent saturation} = \frac{\text{CO content}}{\text{CO capacity}} \times 100$$

For instance, if the capacity for carbon monoxide is 20 ml per 100 ml of blood, and this is a function of the hemoglobin concentration, and if there are only 2 ml CO per 100 ml blood, the quotient multiplied by 100 equals 10 percent saturation. The COHb percent saturation reflects the percent of the hemoglobin combined with carbon monoxide.

The first question to consider is the normal levels of carboxyhemoglobin in normal nonsmoking mothers and their fetuses. Table I shows data from the world literature concerning the concentration of carboxyhemoglobin in pregnant women $(COHb)_M$, their newborn infants at the time of delivery $(COHb)_F$, and the ratio of infant to maternal carboxyhemoglobin $(COHb)_F/(COHb)_M$. There is some variation, depending on the method. We measure CO with a gas chromatograph. The maternal carboxyhemoglobin averages about 1 percent, the newborns about 1.1 percent, with a fetal to maternal ratio of 1.1.[14]

TABLE I. Relation of $[COHb]_F$ to $[COHb]_M$—
Normal Nonsmoking Mothers

Author	$[COHb]_M$	$[COHb]_F$	$\dfrac{[COHb]_F}{[COHb]_M}$
Gemzell et al.[8]	2.02 (SEM ± 0.21)[a]	2.25 (± 0.21)	1.18 (±0.12)
	0.73 (± 0.08)[b]	1.13 (± 0.14)	1.57 (±0.11)
Haddon et al.[9]	1.94 (± 0.61)	1.70 (± 0.49)	0.95 (± 0.03)
Heron[11]	2.6 (± 0.21)	2.5 (± 0.16)	0.79 (± 0.03)
Bjure et al.[1]	1.01[c]	1.15[d]	1.14[c]
	0.76[d]	1.18[d]	1.55[d]
Young et al.[23]	1.57 (± 0.14)	1.61 (± 0.12)	1.06 (± 0.08)
Younoszai[24]	1.2	0.7	0.58
Linderholm et al.[13]	1.20 (± 0.38)	---	---
	0.44 (± 0.14)	---	---
	0.40 (± 0.01)	---	---
Present Study	1.00 (± 0.05)	1.11 (± 0.09)	1.11 (± 0.08)

a and b by different method.

[c]With anesthesia (SEM cannot be calculated).

[d]Without anesthesia (SEM cannot be calculated).

Adapted, by permission, from Longo, L. D.: "Carbon monoxide in the pregnant mother and fetus and its exchange across the placenta." Ann. NY Acad. Sci. 174: 317, 1970.

There are two principal sources of carbon monoxide. The first of these is the endogenous production of CO. Carbon monoxide is produced endogenously from the breakdown of heme pigments in our body. As protoporphyrin is degraded to bilirubin, the alpha-methene carbon atom is released as carbon monoxide. This was first demonstrated by Sjostrand[19] in Sweden. Coburn and his group in Philadelphia have extended the study of CO production.[2,3]

Figure 1 shows the endogenous carbon monoxide production expressed in microliters per hour per kilogram of body weight. The rate in normal men is about 6 microliters per hour per kilo. Dr. Delivoria-Papadopoulos and her

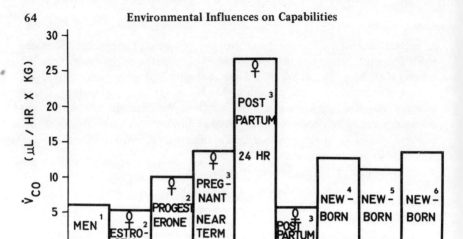

Fig. 1. Rate of endogenous production of carbon monoxide in microliters per hour per kilogram body weight in normal men (3); women during the estrogen and progesterone phase of the menstrual cycle (5); during pregnancy and postpartum (6); and in the newborn [4 = Wranne (21, 22), 5 = Fallstrom (7) and 6 = Maisels, et al. (16)]. Reprinted, by permission, from Longo, L.D.: "Carbon monoxide in the pregnant mother and fetus and its exchange across the placenta." Ann. NY Acad. Sci. 174: 322 c 1970.

co-workers have determined the endogenous production in normal women during the menstrual cycle[5] and during pregnancy.[6] Figure 1 also shows the endogenous CO production in the newborn. Results from Wranne,[21,22] Fallstrom,[7] and Maisels, et al.[16] indicate a CO production rate in newborns almost twice that of the normal adult man. This is probably a reflection of the shorter half-life of the newborn red cells and their higher hemoglobin content. While each of these newborn production rates had been measured with a different technique, they gave essentially the same results.

A second source of carbon monoxide is exogenous, coming from the air that we breathe. Table II shows representative levels of CO in parts per million. Robinson and his group[17] found that the level in uncontaminated sea air

TABLE II. Carbon Monoxide Levels
(Parts per Million)

Fresh Sea Air	0.1-0.5
Urban Air	1-50
Street Corner	5-50
Smoke-Filled Room	25
Major Interchange	100
Auto Exhaust	100-250
Cigarette Smoke	400

is about 0.1 to 0.5 parts per million (ppm). The levels in the Southern Hemisphere at sea are lower than those of the Northern Hemisphere. In the urban air of many of our cities the CO concentration varies from 1 to 50 ppm.

In some parts of Los Angeles during the past year the level of CO has averaged 30 ppm during the day. On street corners the concentrations vary from 5 to 50 ppm. Smoke filled rooms have been measured having 25 ppm. Near major highway interchanges the level of CO is often around 100 ppm. Automobile exhaust has 100 to 250 ppm depending on the car. Pure cigarette smoke has about 400 ppm.

Figure 2 shows the change in the carboxyhemoglobin percent saturation at various levels of CO in the inspired air over a period of time. For instance, if Dr. Behrman's babies breathed 25 ppm they would have just a little less than 5 percent carboxyhemoglobin in their blood after 3 to 12 hours. If they inspired 50 ppm the carboxyhemoglobin concentration would reach 9 to 10 percent.

Figure 3 depicts the relation of steady state blood carboxyhemoglobin concentration to both the carbon monoxide concentration in parts per million and the partial pressure of CO in millimeters of mercury. During the steady state, the fetal carboxyhemoglobin concentration is about 1.1 times that of the mother. This is related mainly to the higher affinity for CO which fetal blood has as compared with maternal blood.[14]

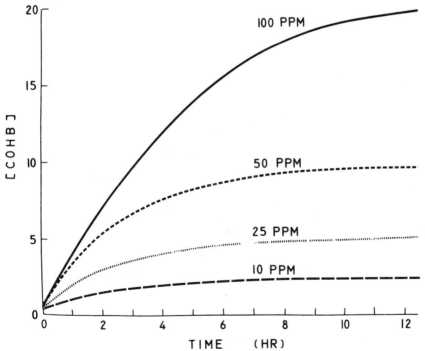

Fig. 2. Carboxyhemoglobin concentration as a function of time and inspired carbon monoxide concentration in parts per million. The curves were calculated from a theoretical analysis (15).

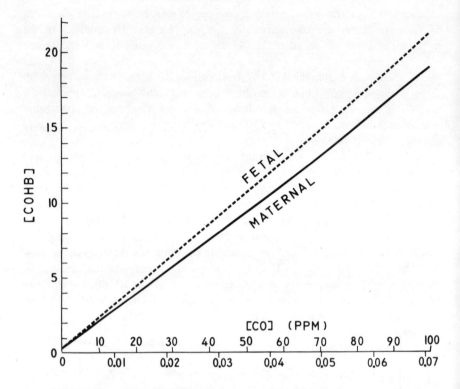

Fig. 3. Relation of human maternal and fetal carboxyhemoglobin concentration to inspired carbon monoxide concentration during a steady state. The CO concentration is given in both parts per million and partial pressure (mm Hg) (14).

What about smoking mothers? Table III shows the reports from the literature. Heron[11] reported mean $(COHb)_M$ of about 6.7 with values up to 14 percent. The mean $(COHb)_F$ was 5, but some values were as high as 12. In our own study, the mean maternal value was 6.3 percent.[14]

The problem with all of these studies, however, is that they were not controlled, either as to the amount the mothers smoked or the relation between the times when the mother smoked last and when the samples were taken. We are now conducting a study, trying to obtain a steady state in smoking mothers. We have found that in one mother who smoked three packs a day, the carboxyhemoglobin concentration was 16 percent in her blood and 19 percent in the baby.

It may also be of interest to consider the changes in maternal and fetal carboxyhemoglobin concentration during the course of a day. Figure 4 shows the change in carboxyhemoglobin of mother and fetus of a "typical mother"

TABLE III. Relation of $[COHb]_F$ to $[COHb]_M$—
Mothers Who Smoke During Pregnancy

Haddon et al.[9]	6.2 (SEM ± 0.75)[a] 3.6 (± 1.06)[b]	7.6 (± 1.14)[a] 3.1 (± 0.84)[b]	1.24 (± 0.2)[b] 0.71 (± 0.14)[b]
Heron[11]	6.7 (± 0.61)	5.0 (± 0.48)	0.75 (± 0.04)
Young et al.[23]	2.0 (± 0.31)	2.37 (±0.30)	1.23 (± 0.08)
Tanaka[20]	5.7 (± 0.24)	5.34 (±0.22)	0.89 (± 0.06)
Younoszai et al.[24]	8.3	7.3	0.88
Present Study	6.3 (± 1.7)	3.6 (± 0.7)	0.73 (± 0.15)

[a]One or more cigarettes 1 hour or less prior to delivery.

[b]One or more cigarettes 1-24 hours prior to delivery.

Adapted, by permission, from Longo, L. D.: "Carbon monoxide in the pregnant mother and fetus and its exchange across the placenta." Ann. NY Acad. Sci. 174: 333 (1970).

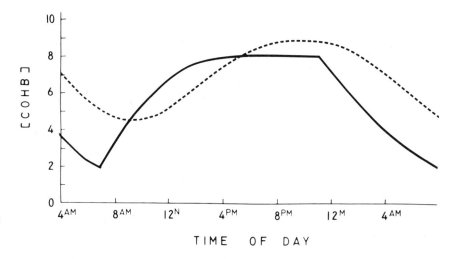

Fig. 4. Calculated carbon monoxide concentration in maternal (solid line) and fetal (dashed line) blood assuming mother smokes 2 packs of cigarettes per day between 7 a.m. and 11 p.m.; or is exposed to about 50 ppm CO during the time period. These curves are calculated from a theoretical analysis (15). See text for details.

smoking two packs of cigarettes a day. The solid line represents the carboxyhemoglobin concentration of the mother and the dashed line that of the fetus. Again, this is a theoretical analysis using a mathematical model.[15] We have some data on the carboxyhemoglobin changes in pregnant women, but we have nothing, of course, on the fetuses. During the night, maternal blood carboxyhemoglobin drops. Assuming that she arises at 7 o'clock in the morning and starts to smoke a total of two packs during the day, that is, one cigarette every 24 minutes her carboxyhemoglobin will rise to about 8 percent by about 1 o'clock and continues at that level. Assuming that she goes to bed at 11 p.m., the carboxyhemoglobin concentration will drop in an exponential fashion during the night as CO is eliminated through her lungs.

The fetal carboxyhemoglobin concentration decreases during the night to about 5 percent. Even after the mother starts smoking, it will continue to drop for a short period of time. At about 10 a.m. it will start to rise slowly and follow the maternal concentration. By about 5 p.m. $(COHb)_F$ will equal $(COHb)_M$. It will be about 9 percent by 7 p.m. and remain at that concentration until about midnight when it will start to slowly decrease. One of the experiments that should be done, now that chronic sheep preparations are available, is to check these theoretical predictions experimentally.

Now the question arises as to the effects of carbon monoxide on the fetus and its oxygenation. Figure 5 depicts the oxyhemoglobin saturation curve of normal maternal and fetal blood.[10] The P_{50}, that partial pressure at which the blood is 50 percent saturated, is 26 mm Hg for pregnant women and about 21.5 mm Hg for the fetus.

The effect of carbon monoxide in fetal blood on the oxyhemoglobin dissociation curve is shown in Figure 6. For some unexplained reason the affinity of oxygen in the blood that is not combined with carbon monoxide is higher and the curve is shifted to the left. One can calculate the effect of different amounts of carbon monoxide in shifting the curve.[14,18]

Ten percent fetal carboxyhemoglobin will shift the P_{50} 5 mm Hg from 21.5 to 16.5 mm Hg. Physiologically, this means that the partial pressure is going to have to drop to a lower level to unload a given amount of oxygen into the tissues. You may say, "Well, the P_{50} doesn't really represent the driving pressure of oxygen from the baby's blood into its cells," and it certainly may not. On the other hand, the P_{50} must be related to the driving pressure.

Figure 7 shows the effects on the P_{50} of various concentrations of carbon monoxide in fetal blood. The P_{50} of normal fetal blood decreases from 20.5 mm Hg at 0 percent carboxyhemoglobin to about 18 mm Hg at 5 percent, and continues to decrease at higher concentrations of carboxyhemoglobin.[15] One of the questions that needs to be considered is how this change in P_{50} affects cellular oxygenation of the fetus and its enzyme systems.

A related problem of tissue oxygenation is the effective lowering of oxygen tension in umbilical arterial and venous blood by carbon monoxide. Figure 8 shows the change in oxygen tensions of the uterine vein and the

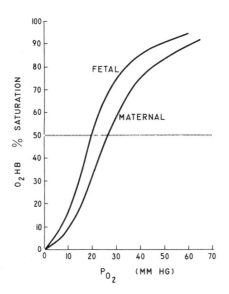

Fig. 5. Oxyhemoglobin saturation curves of normal human maternal and fetal blood at pH = 7.4, PCO_2 = 40 mm Hg, 38 C (10). The P_{50}, partial pressure at which the blood is 50 percent saturated, is 26 mm Hg for maternal blood and 21.5 mm Hg for fetal blood.

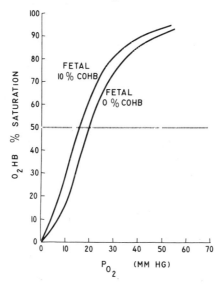

Fig. 6. Oxyhemoglobin saturation curves of fetal blood with 0 percent and 10 percent carboxyhemoglobin. The effect of carboxyhemoglobin is calculated by the method of Roughton and Darling (18). The oxyhemoglobin is that percentage of hemoglobin not bound as COHb.

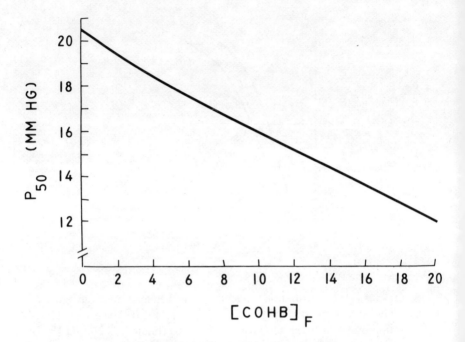

Fig. 7. The fetal P_{50} (partial pressure at which the oxyhemoglobin saturation is 50 percent) as a function of the blood carboxyhemoglobin.

umbilical vein and artery. The normal PO_2 in the uterine vein is around 40 mm Hg. The normal PO_2 of umbilical venous blood is about 30 mm Hg. The umbilical artery PO_2 is around 16 mm Hg. In tissues, the oxygen tension falls to zero in the cristae of the mitochondria of the cells where the oxygen is reduced.

We have calculated the effect of 9 percent maternal and fetal carboxyhemoglobin in lowering the oxygen tension in these vessels.[15] The presence of 9 percent $(COHb)_M$ will effectively lower uterine vein oxygen tension from 40 to about 35 mm Hg. This is because the normal arteriovenous O_2 content difference is increased to maintain normal tissue oxygenation. The umbilical arterial PO_2 will be decreased from 16 to about 13 mm Hg, a 19 percent decrease. This is equivalent to an effective lowering of the PO_2 of the umbilical vein from about 30 to 24 mm Hg, a 20 percent decrease.

(Editors Note: the following discussion was maintained because of the explanatory value.)

DR. METCALFE: Are those calculated values?

DR. LONGO: Yes. In preliminary studies on smoking mothers, we have measured the oxygen tensions. We found that they do not decrease very much. Of course, that is reasonable because within some limits the fetus will probably compensate for any hypoxia with increased placental flow.

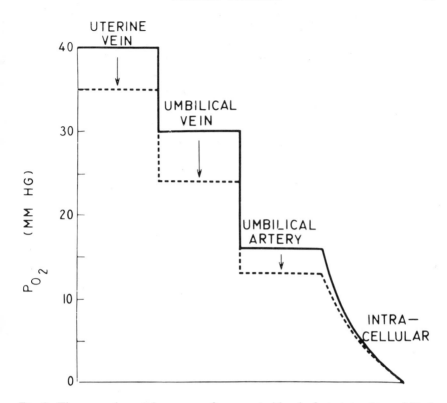

Fig. 8. The normal partial pressure of oxygen in blood of uterine vein, umbilical
vein and umbilical artery (solid line). The effective decrease in PO_2 by 9
percent carboxyhemoglobin is shown by the dashed line. Calculated
from a theoretical analysis (15).

DR. HELLEGERS: Why should it decrease the oxygen tension? I mean,
even theoretically?

DR. LONGO: It lowers the capacity of the blood to carry oxygen. Thus
fetal blood leaving an organ will be less saturated and have a lower PO_2. In
addition, the dissociation curve will be shifted to the left, thus the PO_2 must fall
to lower value to unload a given amount of oxygen.

DR. HELLEGERS: Surely, as long as the mother keeps breathing in and
out, the PO_2 is going to be 100. And why should this decrease the amount of
oxygen per unit area of placental surface?

DR. LONGO: Part of it is that the maternal blood is partly saturated with
carbon monoxide, and the PO_2 in maternal placental end-capillary vessels will be
decreased as the O_2 content will be lower to maintain a normal arteriovenous
difference. The fetal placental end-capillary PO_2 will also be decreased since it
equilibrates with the maternal PO_2.

DR. HELLEGERS: You know, one of the things you could say is the fetus has a greater affinity for oxygen. Isn't that right?

DR. LONGO: Exactly.

DR. HELLEGERS: It is like the to do with bicarbonate. In the future, let's have the mother smoke instead of giving bicarbonate to the fetus. I don't see why increasing fetal affinity for oxygen should lower the PO_2.

DR. LONGO: You are increasing the fetal affinity for oxygen but also decreasing the fetal capacity. The effect is greater than just a decrease in the capacity due to anemia. The effect is compounded, so to speak, because you are lowering the capacity for the fetal blood for oxygen. When you lower the content in inflowing fetal blood, the blood will equilibrate at a lower oxygen tension for a given diffusing capacity.

DR. HELLEGERS: Should it decrease the content of oxygen when you have a higher affinity?

DR. LONGO: Yes, when part of the oxygen content is replaced by carbon monoxide.

DR. METCALFE: There is the effect of anemia. When you increase affinity, you decrease PO_2.

DR. HELLEGERS: For a given saturation.

DR. METCALFE: So if you take the same saturation in umbilical vein, you certainly can calculate lower PO_2.

DR. SEGAL: For a given flow rate?

DR. METCALFE: All other things remain.

DR. LONGO: Of course, the fetus must be able to compensate for this. Otherwise, infants of smoking mothers wouldn't survive.

DR. SEGAL: On the other hand, isn't it true there is work—I am not sure if it is on carbon monoxide—that shows a vasoconstrictive effect on uterine circulation.

DR. LONGO: Yes. Dr. JoAnn Haberman of the Department of Radiology, University of Oklahoma Medical Center is using thermography to measure utero-placental blood flow. In this technique, heat sensors record the heat distribution from a given area of the body. Figure 9 shows a thermogram from a near-term pregnant patient before and after smoking and inhaling from a single cigarette for 8 minutes. The thermal imprint of the placenta (white area between arrows) in the panel on the left, is markedly decreased following smoking (panel on right). While there is an assumption whether this technique measures blood flow or blood volume in a given area, it is evident from these figures that maternal smoking is associated with changes in heat emission from the pregnant uterus. These changes are probably due to nicotine in tobacco smoke rather than carbon monoxide.

DR. HELLEGERS: But the question is whether carbon monoxide has anything to do with the change in oxygen. If you infuse bicarbonate into the fetus *in utero* of a sheep, but never smoke a cigarette, you will lower the PO_2 but the oxygen consumption per kilogram of fetus will remain absolutely constant. I am not sure that when you say simply that you know with smoking

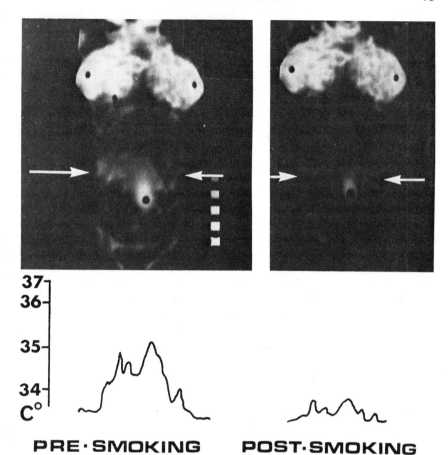

Fig. 9. Thermogram from a near-term pregnant patient before and after smoking. The normal thermal imprint of the placenta is shown on the left as a white area between the arrows. The right panel shows decreased heat emission after the mother smoked a single cigarette for 8 minutes. Below are the temperature profiles across the abdomen at the level of the arrows. The small squares in the left panel are the temperature calibrations. (Courtesy of Dr. JoAnn D. Haberman).

you shift the oxygen dissociation curve to the left, therefore, the PO_2 falls, the implication is not necessarily bad.

I have infused hydrochloric acid into the sheep fetuses and shifted the curve clear over to the right and found that PO_2 increased. There are series of explanations for this result other than carbon monoxide. But a fall in PO_2, will shift the curves automatically, but these have no implications for either the amount of oxygen crossing or the amount of oxygen being consumed. I would not want a national lay magazine to suggest, or a Presidential Commission to report, that, therefore, mental retardation has occurred. I think the explanation is quite apart from carbon monoxide.

DR. LONGO: Carbon monoxide can lower the capacity of the fetal blood for oxygen and change the affinity. In doing this, it can be equivalent to these kinds of changes. These are calculated equivalent changes when given amounts of carbon monoxide are combined with hemoglobin.

DR. BEHRMAN: Dr. Longo is not trying to show that anything has been proved. We were talking about mechanisms and possibilities, suggesting that the process that causes death from carbon monoxide poisoning in high concentration may occur in minimal degree in the maternal-fetal unit, producing tissue hypoxia. I don't think anybody knows the correct answer.

DR. LONGO: Figure 10 shows the calculated decrease in the rate of oxygen change. This is from our mathematical model.[12,15] We have used oxyhemoglobin saturation curves with varying amounts of carbon monoxide—5, 10, 15, and 20 percent. These oxygen exchange rates are calculated from the model, assuming no compensatory mechanisms on the part of the fetus. The O_2 exchange rate decreases almost literally as a function of the amount of carbon monoxide in the fetal blood. Again, I don't think this is happening *in vivo*

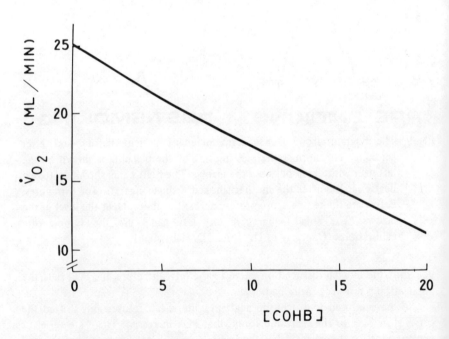

Fig. 10. Decrease in rate of placental oxygen exchange as a function of blood carboxyhemoglobin. Calculated from a theoretical analysis (15) using a mathematical model of placental exchange (12).

because of fetal compensatory mechanisms, such as increased umbilical blood flow.

Coburn and Mayers[4] have recently reported that in man there are shifts in the ratio of carboxymyoglobin to carboxyhemoglobin in both skeletal muscle and myocardium as a function of the oxygen tension (Figure 11). For instance, they find that in normal resting man the ratio of carboxymyoglobin to carboxyhemoglobin will also be 1 percent and myocardium carboxymyoglobin 2 percent. When the arterial oxygen tension is lowered to 40 mm Hg, there is a shift to carbon monoxide into the myoglobin so that the carboxymyoglobin-to-carboxyhemoglobin ratio increases to about 3 in skeletal muscle and about 6 in the myocardial cells.

The fetus never has an oxygen tension greater than 40. We are currently studying whether the amount of carboxymyoglobin in the sheep fetus is as great in relation to the carboxyhemoglobin. If it is, then under normal circumstances with about 1 percent carboxyhemoglobin in the blood, the myocardium will have about 6 percent carboxymyoglobin.

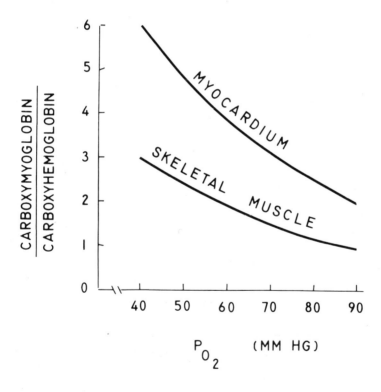

Fig. 11. Ratio of carboxymyoglobin to carboxyhemoglobin as a function of partial pressure of oxygen in myocardium and skeletal muscle in adult dogs (4).

The question arises as to whether additional amounts of carbon monoxide in the blood—say, 5 percent (as the fetus and mother would have when the inspired CO concentration was about 25 ppm, or the mother smoking 1-1/3 packs of cigarettes per day), if the ratio is 6 in the heart, the myocardial myoglobin would be 30 percent saturated with CO.

One wonders what effect this has on oxygenation of the fetal heart under these circumstances.

Finally, there is another piece of experimental evidence on the biologic effects of CO. Tanaka[20] measured the placental oxygen consumption in nonsmoking and smoking mothers (Figure 12) in placental slices in a Warburg apparatus. With tissue from normal, nonsmoking mothers, the oxygen consumption was about 1.9 microliters per milligram placenta per hour. With tissue from smoking mothers, the rate decreased in proportion to the concentration of carboxyhemoglobin in their blood.

One wonders how this decrease in placental oxygen consumption affects placental enzyme systems involved in active transport and metabolism? There

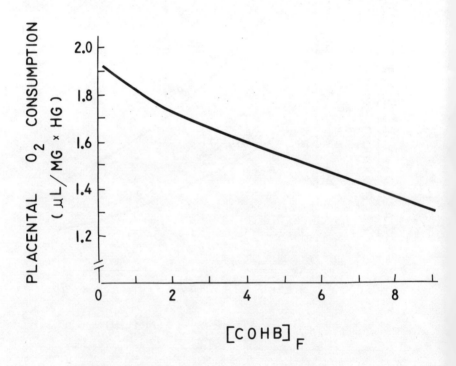

Fig. 12. Measured human placental oxygen consumption (in microliters per milligram placental weight per hour) as a function of maternal carboxyhemoglobin concentrations. From data of Tanaka (20).

are a number of enzymes in the placenta that are very sensitive to carbon monoxide such as cytochrome oxidase, cytochrome P_{450} and carbonic anhydrase. Interference with these enzyme functions may be one of the mechanisms important in the genesis of smaller babies in mothers who smoke during pregnancy.

The other thing, I think, that should be mentioned is that all of these different effects of CO may operate either individually or together to compromise the delivery and utilization of oxygen to fetal and newborn cells. If present for short duration at critical periods or continued for prolonged periods, these effects may interfere with normal fetal development.

There are a number of other questions that need to be explored. To what extent do the decreases in P_{50} affect cellular respiration in the fetus? What is the significance of the shifts of the ratio of carboxymyoglobin to caroxyhemoglobin in cardiac and skeletal muscle? To what extent is the fetus damaged by chronic exposure to low levels of carbon monoxide? Do physical, mental, psychomotor, or perhaps even behavioral sequelae develop as a consequence to the CO levels encountered in air pollution or maternal smoking? What are the threshold levels of CO below which there are no effects on tissue oxygenation? What are the minimal allowable levels of CO to which pregnant women or newborns could be exposed?

Finally, there is another point. As Dr. Behrman noted, we are only looking at one aspect of the air pollution problem. Ozone, the oxides of sulfur and nitrogen and the hydrocarbons may be additional factors that compromise the fetus and newborn. While it is easy to raise these questions, it will be extremely difficult to arrive at meaningful answers. If I may make one suggestion, I think it would be appropriate to conduct a controlled prospective study on the effects of chronic exposure to CO in the development of children of mothers who smoke or who live in regions of heavy air pollution.

BIBLIOGRAPHY

1. Bjure, J., Fallstrom, S.P., "Endogenous Formation of Carbon Monoxide in Newborn Infants. I. Non-icteric and Icteric Infants without Blood Group Incompatibility," Acta. Paediat. Scand., 52: 361-366 (1963).

2. Coburn, R.F., "The Carbon Monoxide Body Stores," Ann. New York Acad. Sci., 174: 11-22 (1970).

3. Coburn, R.F., Blakemore, W.S., Forster, R.E., "Endogenous Carbon Monoxide Production in Man," J. Clin. Invest., 42: 1172-1178 (1963).

4. Coburn, R.F., Mayers, L.B., "Myoglobin O_2 Tension Determined from

Measurements of Carboxymyoglobin in Skeletal Muscle," Amer. J. Physiol., 220: 66-74 (1971).

5. Delivoria-Papadopoulos, M., Coburn, R.F., Forster II, R.E., "Cyclical Variation of Heme Destruction and Carbon Monoxide Production in the Normal Female," J. Clin. Invest. (in press) (1971).

6. Delivoria-Papadopoulos, M., Coburn, R.F., Longo, L.D., Forster II, R.E., "Endogenous Carbon Monoxide Production of Mother + Fetus," Society for Pediatric Research, 39th Annual Meeting, Atlantic City, N.J., May 2-3, 1969, Program and Abstracts, p. 148.

7. Fallstrom, S.P., "On the Endogenous Formation of Carbon Monoxide in Full-term Newborn Infants," Acta Paed. Scand., Suppl., 189, 1-27 (1969).

8. Gemzell, C.A., Robbe, H., Strom, G., "On the Equilibration of Carbon Monoxide between Human Maternal and Fetal Circulation in Vivo," Scand. J. Clin. and Lab. Invest., 10: 372-378 (1958).

9. Haddon, W. Jr., Nesbitt, R.E.L., Garcia, R., "Smoking and Pregnancy: Carbon Monoxide in Blood During Gestation and at Term," Obstet. and Gynec., 18: 262-267 (1961).

10. Hellegers, A.E., Schrueffer, J.J.P., "Nomograms and Empirical Equations relating Oxygen Tension, Percentage Saturation, and pH in Maternal and Fetal Blood," Amer. J. Obstet. Gynec., 81: 377-384 (1961).

11. Heron, H., "The Effects of Smoking during Pregnancy: A Review with a Preview," New Zealand Med. J., 61: 545-548 (1962).

12. Hill, E.P., Power, G.G., Longo, L.D., "A Mathematical Model of Placental O_2 Transfer with Consideration of Hemoglobin Reaction Rates," Amer. J. Physiol. (in press).

13. Linderholm, H., Lundstrom, P., "Endogenous Carbon Monoxide Production and Blood Loss at Delivery," Acta. Obst. Gynec. Scand., 48: 362-370 (1969).

14. Longo, L.D., "Carbon Monoxide in the Pregnant Mother and Fetus and its Exchange across the Placenta," Ann. N.Y. Acad. Sci., 174: 313-341 (1970).

15. Longo, L.D., Hill, E.P., "The Biological Effects of Carbon Monoxide on the Fetus-in-Utero: some Theoretical Considerations," Amer. J. Physiol. (in preparation).

16. Maisels, M.J., Pathak, A., Nelson, N.M., Nathan, D.G., Smith, C.A., "Endogenous Production of Carbon Monoxide in Normal and Erythroblastatic Newborn Infants," J. Clin. Invest., 50: 1-8 (1971).

17. Robinson, E., Robbins, R.C., "Atmospheric Background Concentrations of Carbon Monoxide," Ann. New York Acad. Sci., 174: 89-95 (1970).

18. Roughton, F.J.W., Darling, R.C., "The Effect of Carbon Monoxide on the Oxyhemoglobin Dissociation Curve," Amer. J. Physiol., 141: 17-31 (1944).

19. Sjostrand, T., "Endogenous Formation of Carbon Monoxide in Man under Normal and Pathological Conditions," Scand. J. Clin. Lab. Invest., 1: 201-214 (1949).

20. Tanaka, M., "Studies on the Etiological Mechanism of Fetal Developmental Disorders caused by Maternal Smoking during Pregnancy," Nippon Sanka-Fujinka Gakkai Zasshi (Japanese Ed.), 17: 1107-1114 (1965).

21. Wranne, L., "Studies on Erythro-kinetics in Infancy. VI. A Method for the Quantitative Estimation of Pulmonary Excretion of Carbon Monoxide in Infancy," Acta Paediat. Scand., 56: 381-390 (1967).

22. Wranne, L., "Studies on Erythro-kinetics in Infancy. VII. Quantitative Estimation of Hemoglobin Catabolism by Carbon Monoxide Technique in Young Infants," Acta. Paediat. Scand., 56: 381-390 (1967).

23. Young, I.M., Pugh, L.G.C.E., "The Carbon Monoxide Content of Foetal and Maternal Blood," J. Obstet. Gynaec. Brit. Comm., 70: 681-684 (1963).

24. Younoszai, M.K., Kacic, A., Haworth, J.C., "Cigarette Smoking during Pregnancy: The Effect upon the Hematocrit and Acid-Base Balance of the Newborn Infant," Canad. Med. Assn. J., 99: 197-200 (1968).

Pollution and Infant Capabilities

General Discussion

O. J. Miller opened the discussion by questioning the relationship of smoking to the incidence of malformations in humans. Langman responded that there were no hard data indicating an increase in gross malformations resulting from smoking. Kass then said that the data did show that there was a smaller baby produced by the smoking mother, but, in fact, there was no increase in mortality or morbidity. However, there is a relationship of smoking with sociologic and economic differences among different groups of people. He also indicated that there was a relationship of pollutants, such as that encountered in smoking or in the presence of ozone, to the ability of the lung to clear bacteria. This type of information is under consideration by a number of investigators. The question arises as to whether there are similar effects on the placenta. Segal asked whether the bilirubin-light-machines produced ozone. Kass responded affirmatively, but since there is a considerable amount of circulation of the air in the nursery, the ozone is dissipated.

A number of points were then made by the discussants. Behrman said that it was well-known that carbon monoxide affects nerve conduction time. He wondered how this affects the developing nervous system. Goodwin indicated that she was aware of some data showing a greater frequency of spinal bifida in cases from polluted areas. Kass cautioned that the ability to separate pollution from other various socioeconomic factors, such as urbanization, low income, or poverty, is indeed very difficult. In contrast to the problems outside the home, Sir Dugald asked what of pollution within the home atmosphere. How does this affect the offspring?

Segal summarized these thoughts by indicating that certain aspects of the problem were left out of the discussion of environmental pollutants; for example, mercury poisoning, bacterial contamination, and noise. Certainly, this field deserves considerably more investigation.

Altitude

Introduction

Sydney Segal

If the fetus should escape exposure to carbon monoxide or other pollutants in the intrauterine environment, feto-placental development may be influenced by yet another environmental problem—insufficiency of respiratory gas exchange. This may be imposed by hypercapnia and hypoxemia in the maternal blood stream caused by chronic respiratory or cardiorespiratory disease. There may be hypoxemia alone from maternal cardiac dysfunction. Hypoxemia may be present in the normal woman living at high altitude.

Observations on human reproduction at high altitude will be made by Dr. Jean McClung Goodwin. Dr. Lawrence Longo will also present some of his own material from the physiological viewpoint.

Altitude and Maternal
and Infant Capabilities

Jean Goodwin

Animal studies accomplished over the past 20 or 30 years in altitude chambers and at natural high altitudes have shown that many fetuses fail to survive gestation at such elevations and that those who do, may be small, malformed, or die in the neonatal period.

High altitude includes several kinds of stress such as cold, sunlight, and hypoxia. Hypoxia seems to be the most significant in terms of reproduction. Altitude effects have varied with the degree of exposure. Significant changes seem to require partial pressures of oxygen equivalent to 10,000 feet of altitude. Requirements have varied with species with mice and rats being more susceptible than sheep. Despite this variation, the accumulated data support the conclusion that high altitude hypoxia constitutes a serious hazard to mammalian reproduction.

The first studies of the effects of altitude on humans were done in the mountain states of this country. In 1957, Lichty and his coworkers[8] reported differences in birth weight in hospital populations at different elevations. In Lake County, Colorado, at an average altitude of 10,500 feet, he found a mean birth weight of 2655 g with prematurity defined by weight occurring at the rate of 48 percent of births. Neonatal mortality was 49 per 1,000 live births. The national figures are 3,320 g average birth weight, 7.4 percent prematurity, and a neonatal mortality of 20 per 1,000 live births.

Although in his sample, one-third of the mothers at high altitude were Spanish-Americans, he presumed that racial difference did not affect birth weight significantly.

Because of the severe climate in Lake County, people who live there also had their jobs there. The socioeconomic level is relatively high. The investigators found no difference in diet between mothers having low birth-weight infants and those with infants of normal weight. Lower birth weights persisted even in a series of 111 strictly defined spontaneous singleton infants whose birth had been strictly spontaneous.

One hundred twenty Lake County mothers who had given birth to babies at or near sea level before moving to the 10,000 foot altitude were interviewed. Two hundred ninety-three previous infants born to these mothers at lower altitude had a mean birth-weight of 3130 g. Their 261 infants born in Lake County weighed on the average 2840 g, a mean difference of 290 g. These comparative data, together with the elimination of race, nutrition, and induction of labor as factors contributing to the observed low birth weight, make a strong case for a direct effect of altitude.

Grahn, Douglas, and Kratchman,[4] in 1963, published a review of the effects of high altitude on birth weight in the United States using census data from 1952 to 1957 (Table I). They found a direct correlation between altitude and the incidence of low birth weight. Growth curves of fetuses delivered at different weeks of gestation in the high altitude states and in Illinois and Indiana showed that the effect of altitude on birth weight became apparent only in the last trimester. This timing parallels that seen with small-for-dates infants due to racial and pathologic factors.

The difference in birth weight represented a shift of the entire curve to low values, not merely an increase in the low-weight-classes which would have resulted in a bimodal distribution. They found a highly significant difference of 190 g between mean birth weights in Colorado and those in Illinois and Indiana.

The question of neonatal mortality at high altitudes was investigated in a 1966 study of Mazess[11] in a different setting. He analyzed mortality figures from the 1958 Peruvian census. He found that neonatal mortality in highland departments was 50 or 60 per 1,000, about double that reported for lowland departments. Using the average elevation of the departments, he obtained a correlation of .70 between altitude and neonatal mortality. The number of unassisted births did not correlate significantly with neonatal mortality (Table I).

Mazess conceded that uncontrolled difference in health conditions and

TABLE I. Percentage of Live Births at 2,500 Grams or Less
by Altitude Interval, 1952-1957, Mountain States,
White Population Only. Utah Not Included.

Alt. interval (feet)	Mean alt.	Atm. press (mm Hg)	No. live births	% 2,500 grams or less
0-500	263	753	35,166	6.57
501-1,000	633	743	7,147	6.66
1,001-1,500	1,118	729	73,318	6.17
1,501-2,000	1,786	713	13,809	7.97
2,001-2,500	2,286	699	56,570	7.78
2,501-3,000	2,864	684	12,207	7.14
3,001-3,500	3,256	674	50,933	8.24
3,501-4,000	3,756	662	60,226	8.46
4,001-5,000	4,824	636	100,420	9.47
5,001-5,500	5,237	627	133,617	10.37
5,501-6,000	5,661	617	28,011	9.80
6,001-6,500	6,149	605	53,899	10.74
6,501-7,000	6,767	591	26,619	11.54
7,001-7,500	7,213	582	10,712	11.17
7,501-8,000	7,721	570	9,427	13.04
8,001-9,000	8,519	553	2,474	12.93
9,001-10,000	9,568	532	887	16.57
10,001-11,000	10,410	513	1,697	23.70

Grahn & Kratchman, 1963. Reprinted, by permission, from McClung, J. (now Goodwin, J. M.): *Effects of High Altitude on Human Birth.* Cambridge, Mass., Harvard Univ. Press, 1969, p. 56.

population composition may account for some of the association, but the parallels with studies in the United States suggest that altitude hypoxia itself is an important factor.

In 1966, I undertook a study of birth weight at high altitude in Peru.[10] It was designed to control maternal variables, including race, and data on placental weight and anatomy, as well as infant anthropometry. My study populations were drawn from two Peruvian hospitals, one in Cuzco at 11,200 feet above sea level, and one in Lima at 665 feet. I studied 100 births at each altitude, taking all births within a specified time period and excluding only multiple births and obvious complications, such as toxemia and congenital anomalies. The Cuzco hospital is modern, having been opened in 1965. The Lima hospital is a much larger, older hospital with a daily birth rate of about 100 in contrast to the three births per day at Cuzco.

The Cuzco patients were more prosperous than those in the Lima hospital. Cuzco mothers often said they had come to the hospital as a novelty to see what it was like. Lima mothers often said they came because they did not know or could not afford a midwife.

Fewer than 10 percent of the lower class women in either sample had received any prenatal care.

Results of this study (Table II) showed that at 11,000 feet the neonate was more than 200 g lighter than the one at sea level. However, his head circumference and total length were not less. As a matter of fact, the Cuzco infants were significantly longer. Trunk length, chest circumference, and arm length were slightly less than the mean values for sea level infants. Skinfolds were also slightly thinner at high altitude. The placenta, however, did not weigh less at high altitude. These differences were reflected in a higher placental-weight-to-birth-weight ratio in the Cuzco population.

The relative increase in placental weight at high altitude was apparently

TABLE II. Dimensions of the Neonate and the Placenta at High Altitude (Cuzco) and at Sea Level (Lima)

Variable[a]	Cuzco		Lima	
	Mean	S.D.	Mean	S.D.
Birth weight (gm.)[b]	3,092.8	457.6	3,311.5	479.6
Infant length (cm.)[c,d]	49.6	1.6	48.9	1.8
Crown-rump length (cm.)[b,d]	32.1	1.4	33.2	1.4
Thoracic circumference (cm.)[c,d]	32.6	1.4	33.2	1.9
Arm length (cm.)[b,d]	19.5	1.0	20.2	1.0
Mean skinfold (8 sites; mm.)[c,d]	4.4	0.9	4.7	0.9
Placental weight/birth weight ratio[b,e]	.17	.03	.15	.03
Minimum placental diameter (cm.)[c]	16.2	1.7	15.7	1.7
Placental depth (cm.)[b]	2.2	0.4	2.5	0.5
Cord length (cm.)[b]	43.9	11.4	49.7	9.8
Number of placental infarcts per placenta[c] placenta[c]	0.9	1.2	0.4	0.8
Percentage of placentas in sample with one or more infarcts[b]	53%		31%	

[a]Corrected populations. "Normal" births to lower-class mestizo mothers. N = 73 in Cuzco, 88 in Lima.

[b]P < .01. Difference/standard error of difference = 2.5 or greater.

[c]P < .05. Difference/standard error of difference = 2 to 2.5.

[d]Lengths, circumferences, and skinfolds were taken on only 68 of the Cuzco infants and 85 of the Lima infants.

[e]The Benirshke placental weight, which is the weight of the body of the placenta alone, after cord and membranes have been cut, was used in calculating this ratio.

Reprinted, by permission, from McClung, J. (now Goodwin, J. M.): *Effects of High Altitude on Human Birth.* Cambridge, Mass., Harvard Univ. Press, 1969, p. 80.

accompanied by a slight increase in placental area. The maximum placental diameter in Cuzco was slightly, but not significantly, larger, and the minimum diameter was significantly larger than the mean at sea level. The placenta was also somewhat flatter and more likely to be infarcted at high altitude, and the umbilical cord was relatively short.

A recent study[10] done at 12,000 feet in Peru used a volume measurement to estimate placental surface area. This study also reports greater area of the placentas from the high altitude placentas.

Analysis of maternal variables, including smoking, race, parity, postpartum weight, stature, skinfolds, and age showed that only race and triceps skinfold differed significantly between the populations. It was the Cuzco women whose difference in triceps skinfold was the larger, indicating that they were, if anything, better nourished than the Lima mothers.

The racial difference—Cuzco women being more Indian than Lima women—probably does not affect birth weight. In Lima, the more Indian Cuzco-born women gave birth to infants that were actually higher in weight than infants of the more European Lima-born mothers delivering in Lima. But these infants were 300 to 400 g heavier than babies born of Indian women in Cuzco.

There is additional evidence that the altitude-associated difference in racial composition did not contribute significantly to the observed altitude difference in birth weight. For example, in Cuzco, birth weight was also lower among infants of the more European upper class mothers.

The data elicited several intriguing thoughts. The combined observations from the United States and Peru showed that in both locales, birth weight was lower with increasing altitude. In Peru, this decline was much less pronounced than in the United States. Birth weight in Peru does not reach the value reported for 10,000 feet in Colorado until about the 14,000 feet level. Available evidence indicates that mean birth weight is about 400 g higher in Cuzco at 11,000 feet than in Lake County, Colorado, at 10,500 feet.

Frequency of low birth weight in Cuzco is about 10 percent, less than half that reported at comparable altitudes in the United States. On the other hand, sea level birth weights seem roughly equivalent in Peru and the United States.

Differences in the severity of the altitude effect on birth weight in the United States and Peruvian populations suggest that racial differences, the degree of maternal adaptation to altitude, or factors in the maternal environment may modify the effect of altitude on the fetus.

Studies of Chinese and American Indian births indicate that they maintain high birth weights even under adverse environmental conditions that depress birth weight in other races.

There is evidence that perinatal deaths due to prematurity and to malformations of the central nervous system are less common in Hong Kong than in England. Hong Kong mothers also have a lower incidence of toxemia and eclampsia. The Peruvian Quechua mother may thus have an inherent reproductive advantage over United States whites in addition to her possible specific adaptations resulting from more prolonged personal or racial exposure to high altitude.

Cigarette smoking is the only major environmental factor that would lead to lower birth weights in the United States highland population in contrast to Peru. No regular smoking was found among women in the Cuzco and Lima study samples. No evidence is available on the percentage of women smokers in mountain areas of the United States. However, in a 1964 study of 2,000 births in an urban county in the State of Washington, Ravenholt[13] found that 68 percent of the mothers were or had once been regular smokers. Children of nonsmoking mothers weighed 180 g more at birth than did children of mothers in the highest smoking class.

Mean birth weights at sea level are approximately the same in Peru and the United States, so that unless smoking increases with increasing altitude in the United States, or unless smoking intensifies the altitude effect, this environmental difference could not explain the observed United States difference in the slope of the plot of birth weight against altitude.

A second observation was the absence of infants weighing over 4,000 g at altitudes as low as 6,000 feet in the United States in contrast to populations like that in Cuzco where mean birth weight was maintained at 3,100 g or over. This absence of high birth weight at high altitude may be a more sensitive index of the direct effects of hypoxia on gestation than are increases in the incidence of low birth weight infants.

Little is known about the causes of very high birth weight. Maternal diabetes is a well-known factor. Calderson and coworkers[2] have studied glucose levels in acclimatized women at an altitude of 15,900 feet in Peru. They report below normal levels in nonpregnant women at high altitude and a proportionately lesser decrease in blood glucose during pregnancy at high altitude. Twenty-one women at sea level in the third trimester of pregnancy had a mean glucose level of 69.3, whereas the mean for 12 pregnant women at high altitude was 64.3. The numbers were small, but the authors did attribute significance to these differences.

Low maternal glucose levels could put an upper limit on birth weight. And the extremely large infants associated with maternal hyperglycemia might not be observed at high altitudes.

A third observation of altitude effects was the occurrence of one or more infarcts in 53 percent of the high altitude placentas. Although the diagnosis of infarcts is highly dependent upon the quality of placental examination techniques, the methods were identical in both Peruvian groups. The percent of infarcted placentas from Lima is in the range of 20 to 30 percent of that found in Boston.

Within the lower class Cuzco sample, the number of infarcts per placenta correlated significantly with the mother's race—the more European women having more placental infarcts. As would be expected from this association, the more European upper class Cuzco women had an even higher percentage of infarcted placentas than was found in the lower class: 14 of 18, that is 78 percent, of the placentas from upper class women having one or more infarcts. Placental infarcts leads to a reduction in effective capillary bed which may amount to a loss of one-half of the exchange area predicted from a given placental weight.

Van Den Berg and Yerushalmy[15] report that the percentage of infarcted placentas associated with fetuses with a slow intrauterine growth rate is three times that found in the placentas of rapidly growing fetuses. The presence of infarcts is evidently associated with real impairment of placental function. And the implication of the Cuzco data is that at high altitude such impairment is more likely in European than in Indian women.

A recent animal experiment provides further evidence that placental infarction is increased at high altitudes. Delaquerriere and Valdivia[3] exposed 66 pregnant guinea pigs to simulated altitudes of 13,000 to 15,000 feet. They found massive placental infarcts associated with fetal or early neonatal death in 37 percent of the altitude-exposed animals, as opposed to 6 percent in controls. In this experiment, there was evidence of premature aging of the placenta at high altitude. Fibrin deposition and perilobular thrombi were found in 56 percent of placentas at high altitude and only 33 percent of controls. If the animals were exposed to sudden, rapid ascent to an hypoxic atmosphere during pregnancy, placental infarction tended to be massive and associated with basal hematomas. A more gradual exposure to high altitude showed a tendency to microinfarction.

In summary, we can formulate a consistent picture of the effect of high altitude on human pregnancy. Birth weight is decreased in proportion to altitude. This decrease seems to be congruent with the delayed growth observed in older children at high altitude.

Neonatal and infant mortality increase with increasing altitude. This seems to be true, even allowing for the general decline in the efficiency of delivery of medical care with increasing altitude. Male infants are at higher risk in respect to both the altitude effects—low birth weight, and high mortality.

Although the common causes of altitude-associated mortality and morbidity are not yet defined, we do know that the incidence of patent ductus arteriosus[1,5,9] varies directly with altitude. There are indications that cleft palate[6,7,12] may be also associated with altitude.

Both the placenta as well as the fetus are modified in the high altitude environment. The placenta has a greater weight per unit weight of the fetus, greater surface area, and increased number of capillaries per unit area, as well as a greater tendency to infarction.

With the data available, we can begin to define the high risk mothers at altitude. These would include women who come to high altitude during their pregnancy. Women in the United States are less efficient than Peruvians in maintaining the fetal weight at high altitude. This may be related to the added effect of cigarette smoking which is more prevalent in North American women. The Peruvian mountain women who maintain birth weight when at altitude have larger babies while at sea level than those delivered by women acclimatized to sea level. On the other hand, the Lake County women who show such pronounced effects from altitude had babies at sea level whose weights were still on the low side of normal. Therefore, prior birth weights at sea level may have predictive value in evaluating a pregnancy at high altitude.

Exercise at altitude is a factor known to improve the acclimatization. No one has yet studied whether the extensive herding activities of Andean women during pregnancy have an important effect on the improvement of birth weight.

Another area for future research is the phenomenon of increasing mean birth weight in Lake County, Colorado over the 14 years since Lichty's study. Incidence of low birth weight has declined steadily over this period. What has changed: smoking, race, obstetric management? This remains to be investigated.

There remain many unknowns. Data on birth weight at high altitude were collected before the techniques for amniotic fluid analysis and soft tissue criteria of neonatal maturity had become standardized for the estimation of fetal age. Therefore, we cannot say with certainty whether high altitude affects the time of gestation, or if length of gestation is related either to the birth weight or to mortality effects of high altitude. Evidence available from neonatal anthropometry and from mothers' estimates of gestation time indicates that if altitude affects the duration of pregnancy, the difference is not obvious. However, even small differences in gestational age can alter the appearance of the placenta at birth.

Discrepancies among available accounts of placental anatomy at high altitude may relate to the degree of aging of the placentas that had been modified by altitude.

Ultimately, one would like to identify the high risk fetus at altitude *in utero,* and to apply specific management.

Data from fetal monitoring at high altitude have not yet been reported. These methods, as well as amniocentesis, may first appear as a clinical rather than a research tool in high altitude centers.

If, as some evidence suggests, the high altitude fetus suffers from a deficiency of nutriments as well as of oxygen, it may be possible in the future to bypass the placenta and supply the missing factors, such as glucose, perhaps by infusion into the amniotic fluid. During labor and delivery at high altitude, perhaps the liberal use of oxygen and blood transfusion to the mother may improve the outcome.

If there is a meaningful analogy to be made between the infarcted placentas and small babies seen at altitude and the situation in toxemia and placental dysfunction, early induction of labor may have a place in obstetric management at these upper elevations.

In terms of the management of the newborn infant, more information is needed about the causes of neonatal death at high altitude. The premature baby at high altitude will probably be at greater risk simply because he is also small for gestational age. Further information may show a higher incidence of respiratory distress and may contribute, together with the low ambient oxygen pressures, to the tenfold increase in patent ductus arteriosus[1,5,9] found at 14,000 feet in Peru.

Temperature regulation may be more critical in the hypoxic environment at altitude. Hemoglobin levels of these neonates are reported to be quite variable, but optimal and dangerous levels have not yet been defined.

There is a report that lactating sheep at altitude secrete an erythropoietic[14] factor. However, we cannot yet say whether this should or should not effect the reduction for breast-feeding at high altitude.

In terms of delivery of health care, regions at 10,000 feet and more should be given high priority for one establishment of fetal and neonatal intensive care units. We can now say definitively that some parameters of pregnancy at high altitude are statistically different from those at sea level. It is time now to investigate the pathological cases at high altitude and to determine how these differ from the normal cases.

BIBLIOGRAPHY

1. Alzamora-Castro, V., "Sobre la Posible Influencia de las Grandes Alturas en la Determinacion de Algunas Malformaciones Cardiacas," Rev. Peru. Cardiol. (Lima), 1: 189-198 (1952).

2. Calderson, R., Uerena, A., Munive, L., Kruger, F., "Intravenous Glucose Tolerance Test in Pregnancy in Women Living in Chronic Hypoxia," Diabetes, 15: 130-132 (1966).

3. Delaquerriere-Richardson, L., Valdivia, E., "Effects of Simulated High Altitude on Pregnancy: Placental Morphology in Guinea Pigs," Arch. Path., 84: 405-417 (1967).

4. Grahn, D., Kratchman, J., "Variation in Neonatal Death Rate and Birth Weight in the United States and Possible Relations to Environmental Radiation, Geology and Altitude," Am. J. Hum. Genet., 15: 329-352 (1963).

5. Hellriegel, K.O., "El Ductus Arterioso Persistente: Observaciones Hechas in las Grandes Alturas," Rev. Asoc. Med. Yauli, VIII: 20-31 (1963).

6. Ingalls, T.H., Curley, F.J., "Principles Governing the Genesis of Congenital Malformations Induced in Mice by Hypoxia," New Eng. J. Med., 257: 1121-1127 (1957).

7. Ingalls, T.H., Curley, F.J., Prindle, R.A., "Experimental Production of Congenital Anomalies," New Eng. J. Med., 247: 757-768 (1952).

8. Lichty, J.A., Ting, R.Y., Bruns, P.D., Dyar, E., "Studies of Babies Born at High Altitudes: I. Relation of Altitude to Birth Weight. II. Measurement of Birth Weight, Body Length, and Head Size. III. Arterial Oxygen Saturation and Hematocrit Values at Birth," Am. Med. Assoc. Dis. Child., 93: 666-677 (1957).

9. Marticorena, E., Severino, J., Penaloza, D., Hellriegel, K., "Influencia de las Grandes Alturase in La Determinacion de la Persistencia del Canal Arterial: Observaciones Realizadas en 3500 Escolates de Altura a 4330 Metros Sobre el Nivel del Mar," Rev. Asoc. Med. Prov. Yauli, IV: 37-45 (1959).

10. McClung, J., *Effects of High Altitude on Human Birth,* Cambridge, Massachusetts, Harvard University Press, 1969.

11. Mazess, R.B., "Neonatal Mortality and Altitude in Peru," Am. J. Phys. Anthrop. 23: 209-214 (1966).

12. Pereda, Personal communication to McClung, J.

13. Ravenholt, R.T., Levinski, M.J., Nellist, D.J., Takenage, M., "Effects of Smoking upon Reproduction," Am. J. Obst. and Gynec., 96: 267-281 (1966).

14. Stickney, J.C., Browne, T.L., Van Liere, E.J., *Erythropoetin in Goats at Simulated High Altitude,* New York, Pergamon Press, 1962.

15. Van Den Berg, B.J., Yerushalmy, J., "The Relationship of the Rate of Intrauterine Growth of Infants of Low Birth Weight to Mortality, Morbidity, and Congenital Anomalies," J. Pediat., 69: 531-545 (1966).

Altitude and Maternal and Infant Capabilities

Discussion

Lawrence D. Longo

I shall explore some theoretical limitations of placental exchange by means of mathematical modeling that have been used by Dr. Gordon G. Power, Miss Esther Hill, and me.[3,6,13] This may simulate gas transfer under normal or hypoxic conditions, such as those just demonstrated by Mrs. Goodwin. Such a model can be useful in suggesting further experimental work.

Figure 1 shows a diagrammatic representation of the placenta with the maternal arterial blood coming in, and the uterine vein draining on one side, the fetal blood entering through the umbilical artery and draining via the umbilical vein on the other side. The placental membranes are between these vessels. There are several major determinants to the amount of oxygen exchange.[6] First is the oxygen tension, or partial pressure, in the maternal arterial blood and in the fetal arterial blood. Another determinant is the maternal hemoglobin flow rate. This actually includes both the rate of blood flow and the oxygen-carrying capacity of the blood. The fetal hemoglobin flow rate is also important. Another factor is

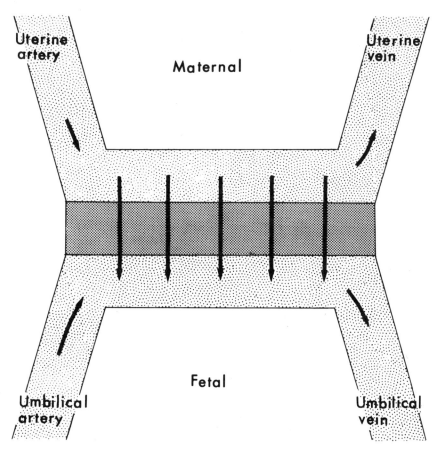

Fig. 1. Diagrammatic representation of maternal and fetal placental exchange vessels with uniform dimensions and concurrent flows. As the blood flows along the capillaries, O_2 diffuses in a one-dimensional plane from maternal to fetal blood.

the diffusing capacity of the placenta, or the permeability of the placental membranes. If the diffusing capacity is high, then oxygen can readily move from maternal to fetal blood. If the diffusing capacity is very low, less O_2 will be transferred. Other important factors are the maternal and fetal hemoglobin dissociation curves, the relation of partial pressure to content in maternal and fetal blood, and the amount of CO_2 exchanging. With the release of CO_2 from fetal blood, there is an increase of oxygen-carrying capacity, the so-called Bohr effect.

The spatial relation of the flow in the maternal and fetal placental vessels is important. Figure 1 depicts a concurrent flow system. One could assume countercurrent, cross-current, or other types of patterns. I plan to describe how one can study the effects of isolate changes in some of these factors.

Regarding O_2 transfer, it would be ideal to measure the changes in oxygen tension and content in the exchange vessels of the placenta during the exchange process. Of course, it is easy to sample maternal and fetal arterial blood. Unfortunately, however, we cannot sample blood in the maternal and fetal placental end-capillary vessels. Uterine venous and umbilical venous bloods are mixed venous samples containing blood that has bypassed the exchange area via shunts, as demonstrated by Metcalfe,[12] and Rankin and Peterson.[17] Some blood is probably going through areas of the placenta with uneven distribution of maternal to fetal blood flows as demonstrated by Power and his coworkers.[15] In addition, some of the oxygen is actually consumed by the placental tissue itself.

Thus, experimentally, we cannot get into the end-capillary vessels to see how a given factor is affecting the exchange process. We can only obtain mixed venous samples. To avoid some of these problems of the real world, we have developed a mathematical model. The amount of oxygen crossing the placenta is proportional to

$$\frac{dQ}{dt} = \frac{A \cdot k \cdot \alpha \cdot \Delta P}{\Lambda} \quad (\ldots \text{Equation 1})$$

Where

dQ/dt = The net amount crossing during a given time period.
A = Area of exchange.
k = Permeability of the membrane.
α = Bunsen Solubility coefficient of oxygen.
P = Partial pressure difference across the membrane.
x = Membrane thickness

The intent is not to complicate the situation with formulas, but Mrs. Goodwin referred to the amount of oxygen crossing in a given length of time. This expression describes the amount crossing as a function of the area and the permeability of the membranes of the placenta.

We can see how at altitude, perhaps, there can be adjustments, such as an increase in area. There is little evidence that the permeability of the membranes themselves can increase.

Another factor that is going to drive the oxygen from the maternal to the fetal blood is the concentration difference. And, of course, the higher this concentration difference, the faster this rate of transfer. At altitude, this concentration diffusion decreases.

Another factor that may be important is the membrane thickness. The amount crossing will be inversely related to the thickness. There is some work by Tominaga and Page[18] in which human placenta cultured *in vitro* showed decreased thickness in the placental membranes, perhaps to facilitate the diffusion of oxygen. This has not been demonstrated adequately.

It seems necessary to present yet some additional formulas. This is to show the series of differential equations used in the model.[3] They are:

$$d[O_2] \, m/dt = -Dp \, (Pm\text{-}Pg)/Vm \, (\ldots \text{Equation 2})$$

$$d[O_2] \, f/df = -(Vm/Vg) \, d \, O_2 \, m/dt \, (\ldots \text{Equation 3})$$

$$1/Dp = 1/\Theta m \, Vm + 1/\Theta f \, Vf \, (\ldots \text{Equation 4})$$

Where:

$[O_2] m$ and $[O_2] f = O_2$ contents	(ml O_2/ml blood) in maternal and fetal blood, respectively
Pm and Pf	$= O_2$ parted pressures (mm Hg) at time (t) in the exchange vessels
Vm and Vf	= maternal and fetal capillary blood volumes (ml)
Dp	= placental diffusing capacity for O_2 (ml/min x mm Hg)
Θm and Op	= diffusing capacities of maternal and fetal blood (ml/ml x min x mm Hg)

Equation 2 describes the amount of O_2 leaving the maternal blood. It is related to the diffusing capacity and the maternal-fetal pressure difference. Equation 3 describes the amount entering the fetal blood. Equation 4 states that the total resistance to diffusion is a function of the resistance of the placental membrane and the resistances of the maternal blood and fetal blood. With about eight equations of this type we can describe the system.

Figure 2 diagrammatically represents the area of placental exchange with the maternal red cell, the placental membrane, and the fetal red cell. The total partial pressure difference is the sum of the partial pressure difference from the maternal erythrocyte to the maternal plasma, the partial pressure difference across the placental membranes, and the partial pressure difference from the fetal plasma to the fetal red cell.[8]

It was formerly believed that the only resistance to diffusion from the maternal to the fetal blood was the placental membranes. From some studies we reported several years ago,[8] we now know that it is not true. About a third of the total resistance to diffusion is actually due to the intracellular hemoglobin reaction rates. This is the reaction of oxygen dissociating from maternal

PARTIAL PRESSURE   DIFFUSION
    DIFFERENCE   RESISTANCE

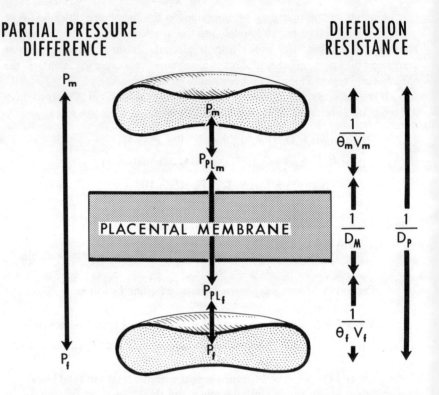

Fig. 2. Schematic representation of the maternal to fetal partial pressure
differences and resistances to diffusion. The total PO_2 difference $(P_m\text{-}P_i)$
consists of: (1) the difference from the interior of the maternal rbc to
plasma $(P_m\text{-}P_{pl,m})$; (2) the difference across the membrane from
maternal to fetal plasma $(P_{pl,m}\text{-}P_{pl,f})$; and (3) the difference from fetal
plasma to the interior of the fetal erythrocyte $(P_{pl,f}\text{-}P_f)$. The total
resistance to diffusion $(1/Dp)$ is the sum of the individual resistances: (1)
the resistance of maternal blood $(1/\theta_m V_m)$; (2) the placental membrane
resistance $(1/D_M)$; and (3), the resistance of fetal blood $(1/\theta_f V_f)$ (see
equation 4).

hemoglobin to diffuse into the maternal plasma and associating with reduced
hemoglobin in fetal blood.

     This is a representation of this exchange process, and shows how the
diffusing capacity is actually a function not only of the membrane diffusing
capacity but of the diffusing capacities of both maternal and fetal blood.

     Figure 3 shows the kind of output we get from this model. Here we have
plotted the partial pressure of oxygen in millimeters of mercury as a function of
capillary length or time in seconds. The upper solid line represents the oxygen
tension in maternal red cells. The lower solid line represents the oxygen tension

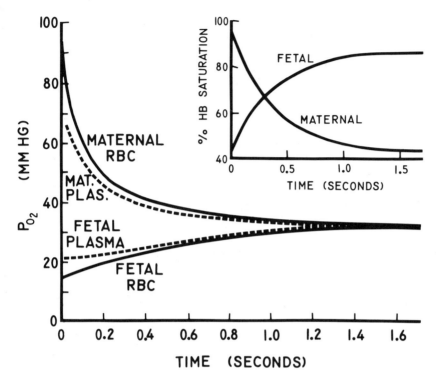

Fig. 3. The time course of change in O_2 tensions during a single transit in
placental exchange vessels. The PO_2 values in maternal and fetal red
blood cells are shown by the solid lines, while the plasma values are
indicated by the dashed lines. Using the indicated values (see text) the
PO_2 in maternal and fetal end-capillary vessels barely reach equilibrium
(< 0.5 mm Hg). The insert shows the change in maternal and fetal
oxyhemoglobin % saturation during the capillary transit. When maternal
and fetal end-capillary PO_2 values are essentially the same, the $\% O_2Hb$
of fetal blood is about twice that of maternal blood because of the
higher O_2 affinity of fetal blood.

in fetal red cells as they approach equilibrium with maternal blood during the
course of a single capillary transit.

We derive this type of a plot from the equations noted above using a
fourth order Runge-Kutta numerical integration technique. We take about 200
steps along the capillary, solving the equations by the forward integration, to
examine the change in O_2 partial pressures and content in the maternal and fetal
red cells.

Taking the hemoglobin reaction rates into consideration, we can also look at the changes in the partial pressure profile of the maternal and fetal plasma. The relative distances between the maternal red cell and plasma is proportional to the resistance of the maternal hemoglobin. The relative distance between the maternal and fetal plasma curves is proportional to the resistance of the placental membranes, while the distance between the fetal plasma and red cell curve is proportional to the resistance of the fetal hemoglobin reaction rate.

This is the kind of plot one obtains. Assuming normal values of diffusing capacity, which we obtained from some carbon monoxide data, maternal and fetal flow rates, hemoglobin values, the values for the parameters in equations 2 to 4, and using this forward integration technique, one calculates that maternal and fetal end-capillary blood will equilibrate at about 31.5 mm Hg.

One of the questions raised was the possibility that the diffusing capacity decreases. From our model and from work that we have done with carbon monoxide, we think that the oxygen tensions are probably equilibrated in end-capillary blood.

In Figure 4 the solid line shows the partial pressure profiles in maternal and fetal blood for a normal diffusing capacity of about 2 ml/(min x mm Hg).

Doubling the diffusing capacity to 4 ml/(min x mm Hg) would result in the maternal and fetal PO_2 equilibrating sooner during the capillary transit. The equilibrated PO_2 values would be the same as the case above, and no additional oxygen would cross the placenta. At least this would probably be true with normal oxygenation. It may not be true at altitude, however, because we know that the mean maternal-to-fetal partial pressure difference is smaller, and the equilibration takes longer to occur.

We have used as many experimentally-determined values as we could, such as the diffusing capacity of the placenta which is about 2 ml/(min x mm Hg).[9] The O_2 partial pressure profiles curves are from the computer output. We are just varying one parameter, in this case the diffusing capacity. (We changed one parameter to see how decreasing or increasing the diffusing capacity would affect equilibration of O_2 tensions in maternal and fetal blood.)

In the model, because we have this one experimental derived data value from our CO work,[9] the pressure profile curves are impossible to obtain, experimentally, under present circumstances. This is because one cannot get into the individual capillaries or exchange units and actually observe how these things are varying during the course of a single capillary transit. Everything I will present is computed using the model.

The model can be used to study changes in one parameter. We will examine its effect on the diffusion process. Figure 5 shows the effects on the mean O_2 exchange rate (ml/min) and the end-capillary PO_2 (mm Hg) as a function of changes of maternal arterial oxygen tension. The dashed line represents normal arterial PO_2 of about 95 mm Hg at sea level. The arterial oxygen tension decrease to 60 mm Hg would be equivalent to an altitude of about 8,000 feet; while 50 mm Hg would be around 11,000.

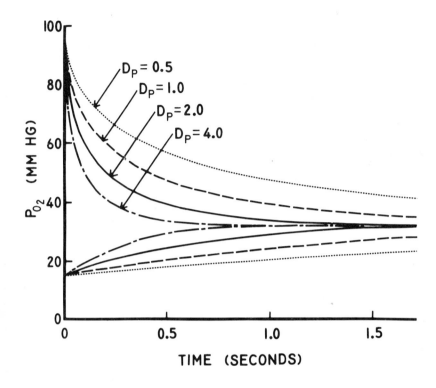

Fig. 4. The change in O_2 partial pressure in maternal and fetal erythrocytes, during the course of a single capillary transit for various values of placental diffusing capacity, Dp. The mathematical model, assuming concurrent flow and normal sheep values, was used for the calculations.

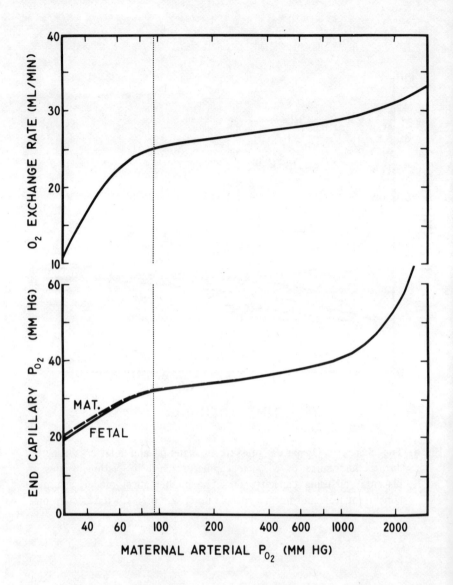

Fig. 5. The effects of changes in maternal arterial O_2 tension on maternal and fetal end-capillary PO_2 and mean rate of O_2 exchange, $\dot{V}O_2$. Moderate increases in maternal arterial PO_2 above normal values (95 mm Hg) increase end-capillary PO_2 and mean O_2 exchange rate only slightly, but decreases in maternal arterial PO_2 produce substantial decreases in O_2 exchange and end-capillary values.

Figure 5 shows that the end-capillary oxygen tension would decrease from about 31 to about 25 millimeters of mercury if maternal arterial PO_2 = 50 mm Hg. This is not to say that this happens in life, because we have compensatory mechanisms. This shows that if PO_2 is decreased and everything else is left on the model the same (i.e., diffusing capacity, blood flow rate, hemoglobin, etc.) this will lower the oxygen tension of the fetal end-capillary blood and actually lower the rate of exchange.

If the exchange rate were to persist without any compensatory mechanism when maternal arterial PO_2 is 40 millimeters of mercury around 14,000 feet, the fetus would die because the amount of oxygen coming to it is less than half of normal.

Figure 6 shows the effects of changing the fetal umbilical artery oxygen tension. As the PO_2 of the inflowing fetal blood decreases, the oxygen tension which that blood is going to reach by the end-capillary is going to decrease. At the same time as the end-capillary PO_2 is decreasing, the oxygen exchange rate is increasing. Intuitively, this makes sense, because the amount of oxygen exchanging is going to be a function of the pressure gradient driving the oxygen across the placenta. As the fetal arterial PO_2 decreases, the gradient increases and more oxygen can cross.

Figure 7 shows what happens with changes of maternal placental blood flow. Again, these are values for the computer run. It has been suggested that at altitude and in other hypoxic states, maternal placental blood flow increases. One can see that with an increased blood flow there will be an increase in the equilibrated oxygen tensions. There is also going to be an increase in the oxygen exchange rate. Of course, the rate of oxygen exchange is going to plateau again because of the shape of the oxyhemoglobin saturation curve. After a certain point, oxygen tension in blood increases considerably, but the amount of O_2 content does not increase and not that much more will cross. This shows that maternal compensatory changes will tend to increase both the exchange rate and the end-capillary O_2 tension.

Figure 8 shows what happens if the fetal placental flow is increased. One might think intuitively that at altitude fetal placental blood flow increases. As the fetal placental flow increases, there is an increase in the O_2 exchange rate. More oxygen can be delivered to the fetus, but as fetal flow increases towards infinity, the oxygen tension in the end-capillary blood is going to decrease, approaching that of the inflowing umbilical arterial oxygen tension. So, in the fetus this compensatory mechanism is advantageous in getting more oxygen across, but works to its disadvantage in that the blood going to the fetus is at a lower oxygen tension.

The cardiac output of the fetus is two to three times that of the adult in terms of unit body weight. This raises the question of how much more work the fetal heart can do.

There may be related compensatory mechanisms at altitude, such as

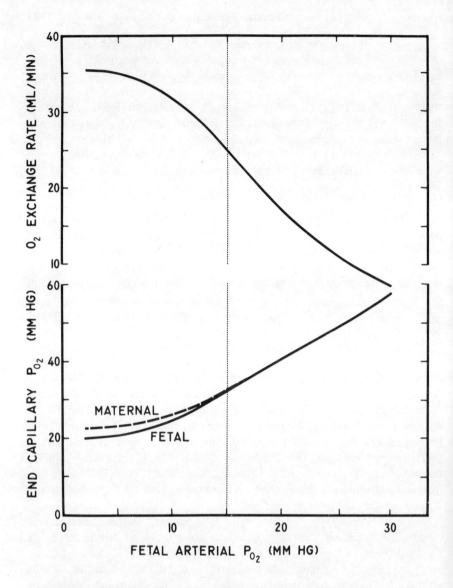

Fig. 6. The effects of changes in umbilical artery PO_2 on end-capillary PO_2 and the mean rate of O_2 exchange. Changes in umbilical artery PO_2 from normal values result in increases in either end-capillary PO_2 or $\dot{V}O_2$, but not both, and may serve to restore umbilical artery PO_2 to a normal value.

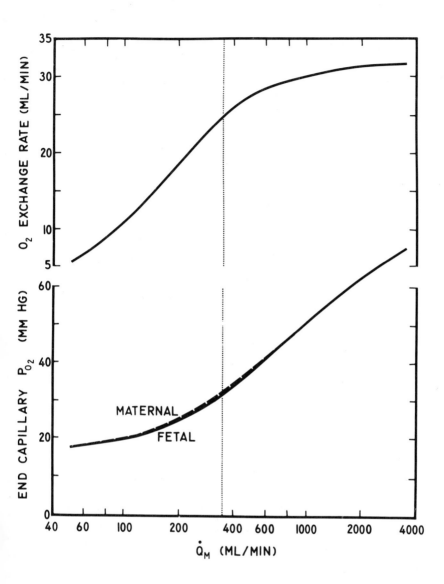

Fig. 7. The effects of changes in maternal placental blood flow ($\dot{Q}_m$) on maternal and fetal end-capillary O_2 tensions and average rate of O_2 exchange.

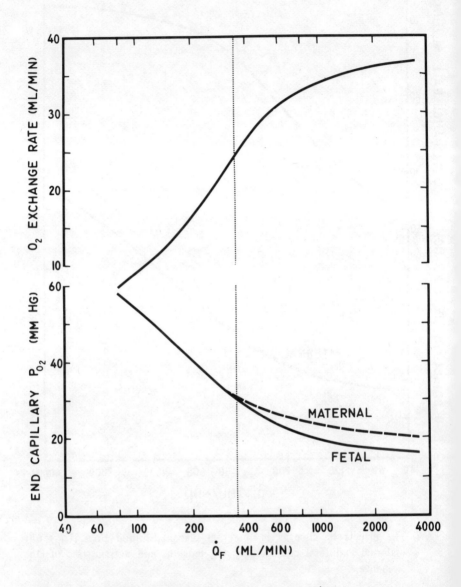

Fig. 8. The effects of changes in fetal placental flow ($\dot{Q}_f$) on maternal and fetal end-capillary O_2 tensions and average O_2 exchange rate.

redistribution of fetal blood flows to critical areas such as the placenta, the brain, and the myocardium, but we know nothing about this redistribution.

Figure 9 shows another possible way that oxygen exchange can be optimized. There is evidence from the work of Power[15] and others of some uneven distribution of maternal-to-fetal blood flow in the placenta. Whether one

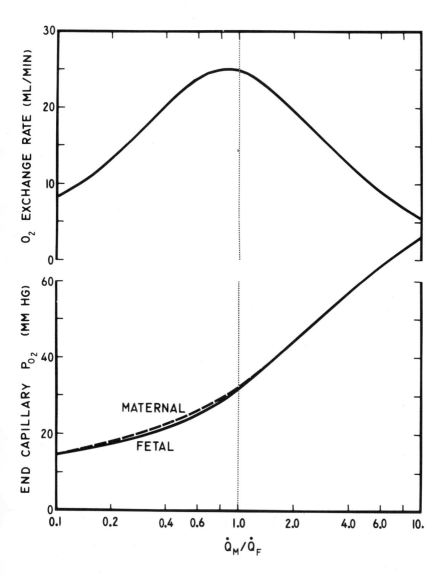

Fig. 9. Effects of changes in the ratio of maternal to fetal placental blood flow ($\dot{Q}_m/\dot{Q}_f$) on the end-capillary O_2 tensions and average O_2 exchange rate. The optimum ratio of $\dot{Q}_m$ to $\dot{Q}_f$ for maximum O_2 exchange is about 0.9.

wants to think of this in terms of vascular shunts where maternal and fetal blood bypasses the exchange area, or uneven distribution, is in a way semantic. The figure shows that the oxygen exchange rate is optimal when the flow ratios are near 1, actually 0.9. Previously, this was shown with another type of theoretical analysis.[14] At altitude, there may be a redistribution of maternal and fetal placental blood flows to make the exchange more efficient. There may also be a decrease in shunting in the placenta. We know from several lines of evidence that there is a lot of shunting. This may decrease. In fact, we showed[15] in the acutely anesthetized preparation that during maternal hypoxia while the sheep were given 10 percent oxygen to breathe, there was a redistribution of maternal-to-fetal flows to make the exchange more efficient.

Rankin and coworkers[16] recently reported that in the "chronic" preparation the distribution of the flow may not be as uneven as we demonstrated in the acute preparation. I understand that Novy and his group in Oregon find a considerable degree of uneven distribution in the primate. This result is still an open question.

Uneven distribution of blood flow is within the placenta. Probably the analogy that more people are familiar with is in the lung where there is uneven distribution of ventilation to perfusion. In the apices of the lung, there is ventilation with little blood flow. In the bases of the lung there is blood flow and not much ventilation. This uneven distribution of ventilation to perfusion in the lung accounts for the so-called alveolar to arterial gradient measured. Even though the oxygen tensions in the pulmonary end-capillaries are identical with those of the alveolus, by the time all of this blood from these different capillaries gets back to the main pulmonary veins, there is mixing. This shows up as a PO_2 difference. This is the nature of the uneven distribution of maternal-to-fetal blood flow in the placenta.

Figure 10 depicts the effect of change in maternal hemoglobin. We know from the work of Drs. Metcalfe, Hellegers, and their group[11] that, indeed, the maternal hemoglobin does increase at altitude. Figure 10 shows that an increased maternal hemoglobin will increase the O_2 exchange rate and increase the end-capillary oxygen tensions.

Figure 11 is a normalized plot where we have plotted how a change in the percent of the standard value, the normal values, for these different parameters affects the end-capillary oxygen tensions. For instance, increasing diffusing capacity (Dp) does not raise the end-capillary tension much. On the other hand, decreasing diffusing capacity below about 80 percent of its normal value lowers the end-capillary oxygen tension. Raising maternal tension (Pm) will not increase fetal end-capillary PO_2 markedly because of the shape of the oxyhemoglobin saturation curve. On the other hand, as Pm is lowered, end-capillary O_2 tension increases.

The slope of these different lines, as they go through the 100 percent value, indicates their relative sensitivity to change. The most sensitive factor to change is the inflowing umbilical arterial oxygen tension. The maternal flow

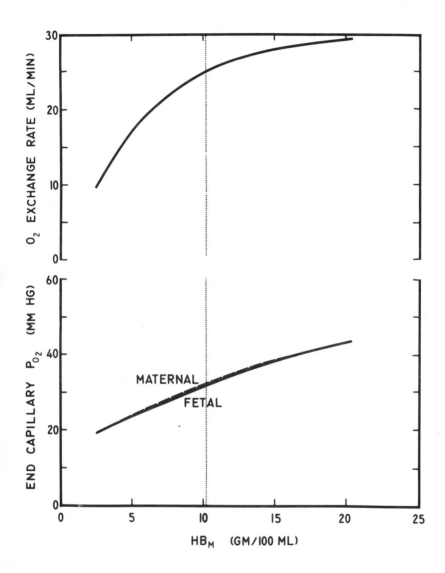

Fig. 10. Effects of changes in maternal hemoglobin concentration (Hb_m) on end-capillary O_2 tension and average O_2 exchange rate. The effects are similar to those of maternal placental flow rate.

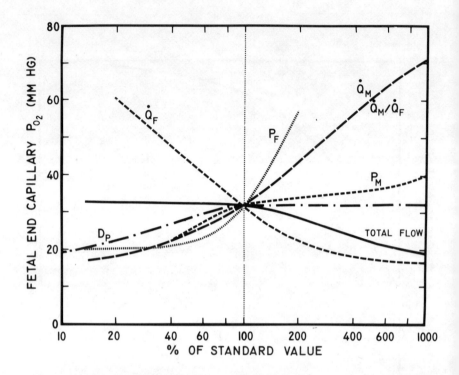

Fig. 11. Effects of changes in various factors on fetal placental end-capillary O_2 tensions. Plot is normalized by plotting fetal end-capillary PO_2 as a function of the percent change of the assumed normal value of a given factor. The slope of each curve at 100% of normal value indicates the relative sensitivity of the end-capillary PO_2 to that parameter. Fetal end-capillary PO_2 is most sensitive to changes in umbilical artery PO_2 (P_f) slightly less sensitive to changes in maternal and fetal hemoglobin flow rates and the ratio of maternal to fetal flow. The curves for maternal and fetal hemoglobin are superimposed on the $\dot{Q}_m$ and $\dot{Q}_f$ curves. P_m and P_f represent the maternal and fetal arterial PO_2 values.

rates, the fetal flow rates, and the ratio of maternal-to-fetal flow are slightly less sensitive.

Maternal and fetal hemoglobin curves are superimposed on flow curves. This depicts the sensitivity of the end-capillary O_2 tension to a given change in the value of these various factors. The last figure is the same type of plot.

Figure 12 shows the effects of changes in the various factors as they affect the rate of placental O_2 exchange. Again, the slope of these curves, as they go through the 100 percent value, represents the sensitivity of the rate of O_2 exchange to changes in the various factors.

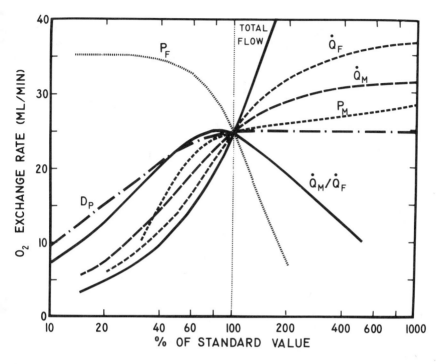

Fig. 12. Effects of changes in various factors on the mean rate of placental O_2 exchange. The plot is normalized by plotting percent change in value of $\dot{V}O_2$ as a function of the percent change in the assumed normal value of a given factor. As in Figure 11, the slope of each curve at 100% of normal value indicates the relative sensitivity of $\dot{V}O_2$ to that factor. $\dot{V}O_2$ is most sensitive to umbilical arterial PO_2 (P_f), followed closely by the total flow and maternal and fetal hemoglobin flow rates. The curves for maternal and fetal hemoglobin are superimposed on the $\dot{Q}_m$ and $\dot{Q}_f$ curves. P_m and P_f represent the maternal and fetal arterial PO_2 values.

Finally, one of the values of this kind of modeling is the simulation of certain clinical conditions. We may examine the effects of chronic hypoxia, assuming a maternal arterial oxygen tension of 50 mm Hg, which one would find at about 11,000 feet.

With no compensatory increases in maternal or fetal hemoglobin, an increase in maternal flow rate of almost 90 percent is necessary for the oxygen exchange rate and end-capillary oxygen tensions to be normal. Of course, *in vivo* the hemoglobin of pregnant women increases at altitude, as does the hemoglobin of the fetus. Using values from the work of Metcalfe, Hellegers, and their coworkers,[11] we find that by increasing maternal hemoglobin to about 16 g per 100 ml blood and fetal hemoglobin to about 18 g per 100 ml, an increase in maternal flow of only 20 percent is necessary to maintain normal oxygenation.

At 14,000 feet, maternal flow rate must increase about 50 percent to maintain normal oxygenation. I think this is probably part of the problem. At high altitudes, these various compensatory mechanisms may become insufficient in a mother who has already compromised herself in trying to maintain her normal tissue oxygenation. This may account for the babies being smaller and not doing so well as normal infants born at sea level.

Another compensatory mechanism, as noted above, is that blood flows in the placenta may become more uniformly distributed.

It has been demonstrated by both Metcalfe and coworkers[11] and by Makowski and his group[10] that there is an increase in the oxygen capacity of the fetal blood at altitude. Behrman[2] has shown that in fetal monkeys there is a redistribution of flows to vital organs such as the brain and myocardium. In addition, there may be an increase in capillarity of fetal tissues. We know, for instance, that in muscles the capillaries are a given number of microns apart. At altitude, the number of functioning capillaries may increase. This would help maintain normal oxygenation by decreasing the diffusion distances for oxygen.

Another possible compensatory mechanism that needs to be explored is the role of fetal myoglobin. Hurtado and his group[4] demonstrated that at altitude there is an increase in the myoglobin content of myocardium, diaphragm, and skeletal muscle.

Little is known about the role of myoglobin in the fetus. There is less skeletal muscle myoglobin in the fetus at sea level than in man. It may be that myoglobin increases at altitude, but the physiologic role of myoglobin in maintaining fetal tissue oxygen tension is unexplored. It may be important.

A related question is the role of each of the compensatory mechanisms in maintaining normal oxygenation at various altitudes and the mechanisms of change as one goes higher.

Nothing is known about the levels of blood oxygen tension that are critical for normal metabolism in the fetus. There are a number of enzymes in the placenta and in fetal cells that require oxygen, cytochrome oxidase, carbonic anhydrase, etc. The placenta is engaged in a variety of metabolic processes, such as protein synthesis, steroid metabolism, and active transport of compounds, such as amino acids. These processes require oxygen, and may be impaired at low oxygen tensions.

We have been discussing the postimplantation or placentation phase of fetal development. What about the preimplantation phase when the blastocyst is still floating free and depending on the oxygen in its environment? To what extent is this development compromised at high altitude?

Dr. Bartels[1] has been doing some intriguing work on preimplantation oxygenation in the sea level animal. This may be a factor in the decreasing fertility at altitude, if indeed fertility is decreased.

Finally, I think that modeling of this type may be particularly appropriate for this conference. This type of modeling shows what can be done with very little hard data, a moderate amount of computer time, and lots of day dreaming.

BIBLIOGRAPHY

1. Bartels, H., *Prenatal Respiration,* Amsterdam, North Holland, 1970.

2. Behrman, R.E., Lees, M.H., Peterson, E.N., De Lannoy, C.W., Seeds, A.E., "Distribution of the Circulation in the Normal and Asphyxiated Fetal Primate," Amer. J. Obst. Gynec., 108: 956-969 (1970).

3. Hill, E.P., Power, G.G., Longo, L.D., "A Mathematical Model of Placental O_2 Transfer, with Consideration of Hemoglobin Reaction Rates," Amer. J. Physiol. 222:721-729 (1972).

4. Hurtado, A., Rotta, A., Merino, C., Pons, J., "Studies of Myohemoglobin at High Altitudes," Amer. J. Med. Sci. 194: 708-713 (1937).

5. Kaiser, I.H., Cummings, J.N., Reynolds, S.R.M., Marbarger, J.P., "Acclimatization Response of the Pregnant Ewe and Fetal Lamb to Diminished Ambient Pressure," J. Appl. Physiol., 13: 171-178 (1958).

6. Longo, L.D., Hill, E.P., Power, G.G., "Theoretical Analysis of Factors Affecting Placental O_2 Transfer," Amer. J. Physiol. 222: 730-739 (1972).

7. Longo, L.D., Power, G.G., "Analysis of PO_2 and PCO_2 Differences Between Maternal and Fetal Blood in the Placenta," J. Appl. Physiol., 26: 48-55 (1969).

8. Longo, L.D., Power, G.G., Forster II, R.E., "Placental Diffusing Capacity for Carbon Monoxide at Varying Partial Pressures of Oxygen," J. Appl. Physiol., 26: 360-370 (1969).

9. Longo, L.D., Power, G.G., Forster II, R.E., "Respiratory Function of the Placenta as Determined with Carbon Monoxide in Sheep and Dogs," J. Clin. Invest. 46: 812-828 (1967).

10. Makowski, E.L., Battaglia, F.C., Meschia, G., Behrman, R.E., Schruefer, J., Seeds, Bruns, P.D., "Effect of Maternal Exposure to High Altitude upon Fetal Oxygenation," Amer. J. Obstet. Gynec. 100: 852-861 (1968).

11. Metcalfe, J., Meschia, G., Hellegers, A., Prystowsky, H., Huckabee, W., Barron, D.H., "Observations on the Placental Exchange of the Respiratory Gases in Pregnant Ewes at High Altitude," Quart. J. Exp. Physiol., 47: 79-92 (1962).

12. Metcalfe, J., Moll, W., Bartels, H., Hilbert, P., Parer, J.T., "Transfer of Carbon Monoxide and Nitrous Oxide in the Artificially Perfused Sheep Placenta," Circulation Res., 16: 95-101 (1965).

13. Power, G.G., Hill, E.P., Longo, L.D., "Analysis of Uneven Distribution of Diffusing Capacity and Blood Flow in the Placenta," Amer. J. Physiol., 222: 740-746 (1972).

14. Power, G.G., Longo, L.D., "Graphical Analysis of Maternal and Fetal Exchange of O_2 and CO_2," J. Appl. Physiol., 26: 38-47 (1969).

15. Power, G.G., Longo, L.D., Wagner, Jr., H.N., Kuhl, D.E., Forster, R.E., "Uneven Distribution of Maternal and Fetal Placental Blood Flow, as Demonstrated using Macroaggregates, and Its Response to Hypoxia," J. Clin. Invest., 46: 2053-2063 (1967).

16. Rankin, J., Meschia, G., Makowski, E.L., Battaglia, F.C., "Macroscopic Distribution of Blood Flow in the Sheep Placenta," Amer. J. Physiol., 219: 9-16 (1970).

17. Rankin, J.H.G., Peterson, E.N., "Application of the Theory of Heat Exchangers to a Physiological Study of the Goat Placenta," Circulation Res., 24: 235-250 (1969).

18. Tominaga, T., Page, E.W., "Accommodation of the Human Placenta to Hypoxia," Amer. J. Obstet. Gynec., 94: 679-691 (1966).

Altitude and Maternal and Infant Capabilities

General Discussion

Dr. Kretchmer opened the discussion by asking Goodwin whether there was a racial difference between the people in Cuzco who were Indian and the women in Lima who were more predominantly European. Goodwin responded by saying that she took this problem into consideration. Although the variability of the data was rather complicated, she believed that the way the data were handled, the racial factors were eliminated.

Behrman suggested that the discussion during the presentation of the papers in this section had indicated that investigators of placental and fetal physiology were attracted to studies of altitude in order to understand maternal-fetal mechanisms in a natural setting. He believed there was relatively little primary interest in whether those women living at high or low altitudes gave birth to high or low birth-weight babies. He urged that groups interested in studies of high altitude physiology concentrate on the identification of the questions that were primarily important to perinatology. Segal suggested the possibility that the low birth-weight infant of the high altitude mother could be viewed as an advantageous adaptation to the environment. Perhaps high altitude gives the opportunity to study the processes of adaptation more completely.

Hellegers indicated that the altitude studies were broadly based and that many of our concepts concerning the effects of high altitude were still only assumptions. Goodwin thought that the clinical situation encountered at high altitude still required considerable study by clinicians, and that participation by this group could be of general benefit.

Kaiser suggested that it would be very useful to determine whether there is a critical level at which altitude begins to affect the size of the fetus. To illustrate this point, he suggested that the perinatal mortality rate at the altitude of the Rocky Mountains-Sierra Nevada Intermountain Region was much lower than adjacent states where the altitude was lower. Kass responded by indicating that Brown and Katchman reported that the incidence of low birth weight in 1,000 live births increased from 6.7 at an altitude under 1,000 feet to an incidence of 23.7 at an altitude between 10,000 and 11,000 feet. He also referred to the Lake County neonatal mortality figure of 41.6 per 1,000 live births in contrast to 23.4 at the Denver elevation. Kass believed that there was evidence of a continuously graded variable in the effects of altitude and urged that these studies be considered with a multifactorial analysis. He added that decreased atmospheric pressure, increased cosmic and ultraviolet radiation, decreased temperature and humidity, and the tendency for people at high altitude to live in smaller houses are potentially important factors. Rossi said that in studies in Switzerland the birth rate was the same at various altitudes. Sereni indicated that there was a large gap between what the group was saying about the effects of altitude and the measurement of the supply of oxygen to the fetus. He suggested that one area of investigation might be in determining the ability of fetal tissues to adapt to low oxygen tensions. He indicated that there was a paper published some years ago concerning tryptophan pyrrolase, which showed that the enzymatic activity changed quite markedly in the presence of decreased oxygenation during fetal life. He went on to say that the brain would be a most important organ to study. Hellegers supported Sereni's comment and indicated that a study was being formed in Holland concerned with the outcome of children of mothers with congenital heart disease.

Minkowski supported the potential role played by environmental temperature on the development of the fetus. He said that there were data from Boston where a number of skeletal anomalies had been reported in pregnant animals exposed to a simulated high altitude. Segal supported this statement but indicated that the simulated altitudes were extremely high.

Sir Dugald was very interested in the problems in the State of Utah where there is an extremely low fetal mortality, even with a large family. Kaiser indicated that the two states in the United States with the highest infant birth rate were Utah and Mississippi, and that there was a considerable difference in the infant mortality between them. Sir Dugald made a classic statement which was, "If you are going to have 10 children for a low mortality rate, then you have to have what it takes." He agreed that in the Southern States an entirely different situation existed than what was present in Utah.

Metcalfe brought up some interesting data indicating that in Laroya, which is at an elevation of 10,500 feet, the incidence of myocardial infarction is very low. Even though the people living in this area are predominantly young and have poor nutrition, they still have a low rate of myocardial infarction. He extrapolated from these data to indicate that maybe high altitude has a good effect on the long-term health course of the infant. He brought up the rather provocative point that low oxygen tension may in fact be good and not bad. "Hypoxia at the time of gestation may in fact pay big dividends in tissue capillarity as well as development of tissue enzymes." He proposed that there must be a series of various adaptations and survivals existing among infants who are conceived who cannot tolerate high altitudes and those infants who can. He said that the human may be much more flexible in his ability to respond to environment than many of us think.

In discussion of Longo's paper, Hellegers indicated that we must distinguish very carefully between the acute lowering of the PCO_2 and the chronic type which exists in residents at a high altitude. This difference between acute and chronic adaptation to hypoxia may indeed be very critical. He thought that the figure set by Goodwin of 10,000 feet was rational. In fact, Hellegers said that he always advises pregnant women not to go above that height. There were some important practical considerations, i.e., that a pregnant woman with tetralogy of Fallot should be advised not to fly in airplanes, since flight will be at an equivalent of 15,000 feet and may have considerable hypoxia.

O. J. Miller discussed the need to define the high-risk mother in relation to effects of altitude. He continued and said that with various genetic problems, such as sickle cell anemia, a pregnant woman could respond adversely to high altitude. Consequently, identification of these genetic problems would serve as a basis for preventive care. One should question whether it is true that the critical factor at high altitudes is a diminished content of oxygen, or whether there are other factors determining production of the small-for-dates infant. O. J. Miller cautioned that consideration of socioeconomic factors was generally ignored in the preceding discussion although we all know that they demand attention.

Genetic and Chemical Influences on Development

Introduction

Joseph Dancis

Genetics is in a very fortunate position at present. The available concepts and techniques have brought us to the threshold of breath-taking scientific opportunities. One question that must be considered is what are likely to be the most profitable directions of investigation to emphasize? The area which we must cover in this session is so broad that it will not be possible to delve deeply into any one subject. Four qualified people will speak on subjects they consider important.

Genetics, A General Statement

Leon Rosenberg

I would like to begin this discussion of the influence of genetics on research in perinatal biology by quoting statistics that have been compiled by some leading geneticists. Dr. James Neel pointed out recently that the estimates of the rates of human mutation per genetic locus per generation are in the ranges of 1 x 10^{-5}. If one assumes that the human genome contains enough DNA to code for 7 x 10^6 polypeptides and that only 10 percent of this DNA is functional, the total mutation rate per gamete would be 7 x 10^5 times 1 x 10^{-5} or 7. This very large number emphasizes the great potential that mutational events have in the regulation of the processes under discussion at this meeting. It also provides a theoretical base for the numerous inborn errors of metabolism and specific cytogenetic abnormalities that we, as geneticists, consider daily.

Additional statistical information from population surveys estimates that 0.5 percent of all newborns in this country have major cytogenetic abnormalities and that an equal fraction have inherited biochemical disorders. These figures suggest that perhaps 20,000 children per year are born in the United States with major chromosomal or biochemical disorders. Professor Joshua Lederberg went even further in his testimony before Congress last year when he suggested that, based on information from Canada and Europe, congenital or hereditary diseases were the second major cause of death in children between the age of 0-5 years, and that such congenital or hereditary diseases were responsible for 25 percent of all hospital bed occupancy in the United States.

If we leave these broad generalizations and think about specific diseases, these figures indicate that there are approximately 3,000 to 4,000 new patients with Down's syndrome born per year; another 2,000 to 3,000 patients with cystic fibrosis; perhaps 500 patients with phenylketonuria; and finally, 20,000 blacks with sickle cell trait. These conditions are some of the most common chromosomal or biochemical disorders, but they account for only a small fraction of the genetic disease in the population.

These numbers give some idea of the magnitude of the problem for perinatal biology posed by congenital or hereditary diseases. I would now like to identify the questions for science and for society posed by these disorders. I do not propose to answer these questions, nor am I going to present any new data. I am not going to discuss any disease at length, but will, instead, try to pose questions in three areas: mechanisms of hereditary disease; detection of inherited disorders; and prevention and treatment of inherited diseases.

The fundamental question about hereditary mechanisms which we must begin to answer in the next decade concerns mammalian differentiation. How is the developmental diversity of cells, tissues, and organs regulated in the face of a common cellular genome? We have very little information about this process, but we do recognize the enormous significance that differentiation has in the regulation of human biology. Nuclear and cytoplasmic factors surely regulate cellular differentiation in man, but we must rely on experiments in nonmammalian organisms for our current data.

Every daughter cell is provided with genetic information identical to that contained in the parent cell. Identification of chromosome puffs in drosophilia and chromosome loops in the newt demonstrate that differential RNA synthesis occurs at different times and in different places along chromosomes, thus highlighting nuclear differentiation as a control mechanism. We know also from nuclear transplantation experiments in frog eggs that the nucleus differentiates. The blastula nucleus is pluripotential and will lead to the development of a normal frog when transplanted to enucleated eggs. However, if such transplantation is delayed until the embryonic nucleus is in the gastrula phase, the resultant frog will have major developmental anomalies. This indicates that nuclear control of organ development is a programmed function.

Other studies indicate that cytoplasmic as well as nuclear factors control the process of differentiation. This is not surprising when we consider that, although the nuclear information in daughter and parent cell is identical, the cytoplasmic information provided each daughter cell is certainly not identical to that found in the parent cell. The experiments which demonstrate such cytoplasmic control have been reviewed by many workers and will not be discussed further.

Let us think for a moment about the biochemical events which must be considered in the process of differentiation. If we start with the genes in the DNA of a fertilized ovum and think about the growth of the embryo, we can recognize several levels of information which are needed. First, we must learn how the information in DNA regulates RNA synthesis, which, in turn, regulates the synthesis of specific enzymes which finally determine the chemical potential of a differentiated cell. In addition, we must begin to consider the many ways in which the intrauterine environment may affect the developmental process. Many of the topics we have been considering during the past two days, such as oxygen availability, nutrients, and pollutants must impinge upon the normal development sequence; yet, at the present time, we know essentially nothing about the molecular interrelations between the intrinsic heredity of the developing organism and its environment.

There are many possible schema by which specific genes can be selectively turned on or off in a cell. I am sure that these processes will turn out to be very complicated and may differ considerably between cells and even within the same cell. One model which has been presented in the literature is based on the Jacob-Monod inducer-repressor system as defined in microorganisms. This theory suggests that differentiation may be regulated by a complex interaction between regulator genes, repressor proteins, and inducer molecules. Such schemes can provide almost infinite variability of sequential gene function, and this flexibility makes the theory attractive. At present, such schemata exist only in the mind of the scientist. They have not been tested in any mammalian systems.

An understanding of cellular differentiation is only one of several fundamental unanswered questions concerning hereditary mechanisms. Information about the localization of human genes on specific chromosomes is very limited. The unique inheritance pattern of X-linked traits has facilitated localization of more than 60 loci to the X chromosome, but only one other 3-point localization has been described in human chromosomes. The loci for Duffy blood group substance, congenital cataracts, and for "uncoiler" are found on chromosome 1. The loci for ABO blood groups, the nail-patella syndrome, and adenylate kinase activity have also been shown to be linked, but the chromosome which carries these genes is unknown. Several other 2-point linkage groups have been defined, but at the present time we can localize only 12 or 13 autosomal genes out of the estimated thousands of genes found on these chromosomes. There is reason to believe that knowledge about gene localization will have application to genetic counseling, but the magnitude of the clinical relevance of this subject will become clearer only with additional information.

A third question about hereditary mechanisms is much more relevant to human disease. The Down's syndrome phenotype is associated with trisomy 21 and is presumably caused by the extra chromosome, but we know nothing about the biochemical events which relate the chromosome abnormality to the particular phenotypic aberrations. Numerous theories exist about specific biochemical abnormalities related to the Down's phenotype, but none of these appear to convincingly relate the genotype to the phenotype. In fact, the extent of our knowledge about biochemical mechanisms of specific inborn errors of metabolism is not significantly greater than that for chromosomal abnormalities. We are beginning to learn a great deal about the specific enzymatic defects responsible for diseases like phenylketonuria, maple syrup urine disease, or galactosemia. In no instance do we have conclusive pathophysiologic relationships between the enzymatic defect and the mental retardation, repeated episodes of acidosis, or growth failure which are seen in the above disorders.

I believe that there are some equally significant questions about hereditary mechanisms with which society as a whole must grapple. The question of national priorities for scientific research has been discussed and bemoaned often enough. I would like to ask whether the organization of our scientific institutions is optimal for the study of the hereditary mechanisms I have just discussed. I believe firmly in nondirective research and in the NIH peer review system, but I also believe that we may reach a point in our understanding of specific diseases at which a coordinated effort by scientists with different kinds of expertise may hasten detailed understanding. Let me take cystic fibrosis as an example. Several recent investigations have demonstrated macromolecular serum factors which affect sodium transport or ciliary action. Other studies have shown accumulation of metachromatic staining material in fibroblasts of patients with this disease. It seems likely to me that a concerted effort by molecular biophysicists, cell biologists, membrane biochemists, geneticists, and pediatricians might help us understand the relationships between these varied observations and, perhaps, elucidate the fundamental mechanism of this common inborn error of metabolism.

The second major area that I would like to touch upon concerns genetic disease detection and prevention. Here again, there are scientific as well as societal questions. Neonatal screening for phenylketonuria is prescribed by law in most states in this country. But there are several other biochemical diseases which lend themselves to such a screening approach. These diseases include maple syrup urine disease, homocystinuria, galactosemia, glucose-6-phosphate-dehydrogenase deficiency, and sickle cell trait. Very few states require screening for these diseases. Economic factors seem to play an important part in the decision concerning which diseases will be routinely screened, but we lack a national policy which relates technical feasibility, disease impact, and economic considerations.

As we define a national approach to neonatal screening for metabolic diseases, we must also consider recent evidence indicating that certain biochemical and chromosomal disorders can be detected *in utero*. There is no longer any doubt that major chromosomal abnormalities and perhaps a dozen biochemical diseases can be detected from examination of cells collected from the amniotic fluid during the first 12-16 weeks of gestation. Increasing numbers of such amniocenteses are being carried out in an ever increasing number of laboratories. Published information suggests that the procedure is safe, but larger surveys are needed to insure the safety of the procedure as well as to define its efficacy as an antenatal diagnostic approach.

Society has a right to ask how these neonatal or antenatal diagnostic procedures are to be organized. Should such screening be carried out by individual laboratories, regional laboratories, central facilities with broad scientific expertise, or should the federal government prepare and support a national policy for such screening? Equally important questions concern the individual patient and family involved in such screening programs. My own recent experience indicates that such medico-legal questions as confidentiality between doctor and patient and the Hippocratic tradition in which a physician defines his responsibility to the patient who seeks his attention are not defined by our current screening programs and must concern all of us who work in the field of human genetic disease detection.

Finally, let me say a few words about treatment. As our understanding of genetic diseases increases, we will continue to extend approaches aimed at modifying the mutant phenotype by replacement of missing enzymes, by replacement of missing products, by dietary limitations, by cofactor replacements, or by surgery. We must also be prepared to grapple with the more complicated questions of genotypic modification, euphemistically referred to as "genetic engineering." I feel certain that directed viral transduction and artificial fertilization with subsequent reimplantation are techniques soon applicable to families with inherited diseases. I will not discuss the specter of cloned human populations. I hope and believe that these techniques will be used for specific patient care with the same prudence that physicians have always tried to use in mitigating human disease.

Chemical Factors Influencing Development of the Fetal Brain

Jan Langman

From Sir Dugald's presentation, it is evident that a considerable number of cases of perinatal death result from malformations of the central nervous system, and throughout this conference anencephaly has been mentioned as an important cause of death. Unfortunately, little is known about the factors causing this abnormality in man. Only recently have experimental teratologists been able to identify a number of factors which cause anencephaly in the mammalian embryo,[11,15,16,18,20,21,31,33,41,42] and the morphogenesis of this malformation has been described.[19,28] A number of conclusions may be drawn from this work: (1) Anencephaly can be produced by a large number of teratogenic factors, but these factors have little in common. When the embryo is affected by a teratogenic agent at a specific time of development, that is, the period during which the neural groove closes, the neural tube fails to close and results in the formation of rachischisis and/or anencephaly. (2) Contrary to what was previously accepted, the central nervous system consists, during closure of the neural groove, only of one cell type, the neuroepithelial cell, and neurons and glia cells are not yet formed.[24]

After the neural groove has closed, the neuroepithelial cells give rise to

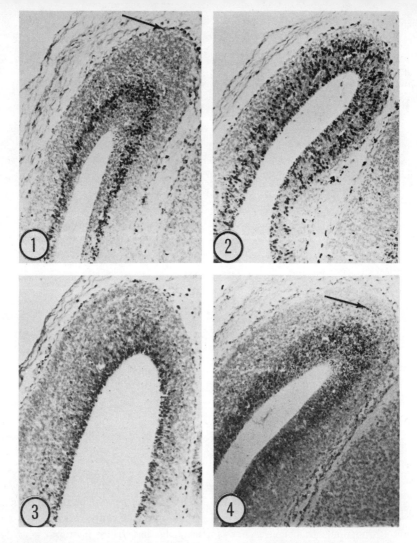

PLATE 1

1 Radioautograph of a coronal section through the cerebral hemisphere of a 14-day mouse embryo one hour after treatment with tritiated thymidine (X100). The labeled nuclei are almost exclusively found in the outer portion of the neuroepithelial layer surrounding the lumen of the lateral ventricle. An occasional labeled nucleus is seen in the mantle layer, but these nuclei are always associated with blood vessels. The pia (arrow) contains many DNA-synthesizing cells.

2 Radioautograph of a coronal section through the cerebral hemisphere of a 14-day mouse embryo four hours after treatment with tritiated thymidine (X100). Many of the labeled nuclei in the neuroepithelial layer are now adjacent to the lumen of the ventricle where they undergo mitosis.

3 Radioautograph of a similar section as in Figure 2 six hours after treatment

neurons and glia cells.[24,25,27] This raises the question of whether teratogenic factors, which are able to interfere with the metabolism of the neuroepithelial cells during closure of the neural groove, are also able to interfere with these cells when they are producing neurons and glia cells at later stages of development. For example, can trypan blue[15,20,42] and dimethylsulfoxide,[16] compounds causing anencephaly when given early during gestation, interfere with the neuroepithelial cells later in gestation and possibly produce neuronal deficits or abnormally differentiating neurons. During the last three years, we studied whether teratogenic factors causing anencephaly when given early during gestation cause more subtle cytological abnormalities when given late in gestation. Thus far we have been unable to detect any cytological abnormalities. In the course of this work it became evident that our understanding of cell proliferation, migration, and differentiation was far from satisfactory. It may be that we failed to detect cytological abnormalities or a neuronal deficit in certain areas of the cortex simply because of insufficient knowledge of the developing cortex. Influence of teratogenic factors on the brain during later stages of development can be investigated by studying in detail the production, migration, and differentiation of neurons. When the knowledge is available, it might be possible to study the effect of various environmental influences, such as malnutrition, LSD, and pollutants on the development of the central nervous system in a much more systematic manner.

To examine in which cells of the developing neocortex DNA-synthesis occurs, 14-day pregnant mice were injected with tritiated thymidine.[29] The animals were sacrificed one hour after injection and the position of the DNA-synthesizing cells in the brain of the embryo examined by the radioautographic technique. Figure 1 shows that DNA synthesis in the cortex is restricted to a broad band of cells surrounding the lumen of the lateral ventricle. With the exception of an occasional labeled cell related to blood vessels, none of the other cells in the cortex contains any label. As is evident from Figure 1, the labeled cells are located at some distance from the lumen. Bordering the lumen are found many dividing cells. When similarly treated embryos were sacrificed four hours after injection with tritiated thymidine, many of the mitotic cells

with tritiated thymidine (X100). The vast majority of the labeled nuclei are located along the lumen of the ventricle and only a few of the labeled nuclei are still in the DNA-synthetic zone (see Fig. 1). The mitotic figures are found exclusively along the surface of the ventricle and all are labeled.

4 Radioautograph of a similar section as in Figure 2, but 11 hours after treatment with tritiated thymidine (X100). The total number of labeled nuclei is approximately twice that seen in Figure 1. The great majority are located in the neuroepithelial zone, but a few labeled cells have migrated into the mantle layer (arrow). The cells containing these labeled nuclei are considered to be neuroblasts.

Reprinted, by permission, from Langman, J. and Welch, G. W.: "Excess vitamin A and development of the cerebral cortex." J. Comp. Neur. 131: 15-26, 1967. (Courtesy of The Wistar Press.)

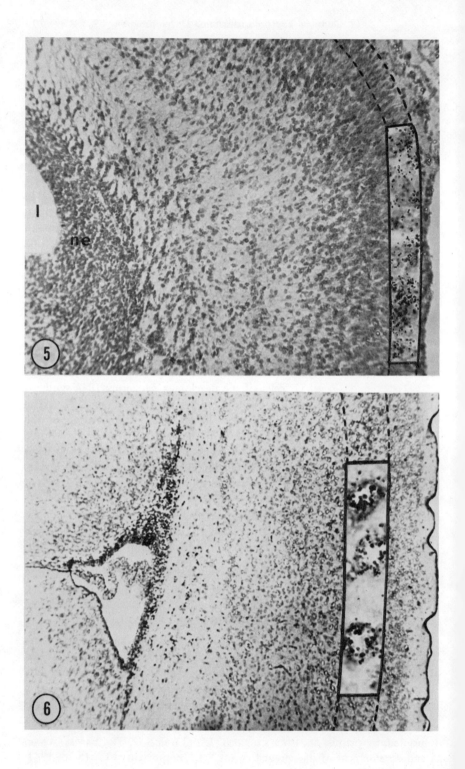

bordering the lumen were found to be labeled (Fig. 2). Since tritiated thymidine is available for incorporation into the DNA molecule for approximately one hour after injection[12,32] it may be concluded that the cells synthesizing DNA at some distance from the lumen have migrated from the DNA synthetic zone to the lumen to undergo division. From electron microscopic studies[14] it has recently become evident that the cells, when synthesizing DNA, are connected to the lumen by a slender cytoplasmic process. When the cell is ready for mitosis, the nucleus moves to the lumen and the cell contracts. Six hours after injection most of the labeled nuclei are crowded along the lumen and only a few remain in the DNA synthetic zone (Fig. 3). During the following hours, the majority of the labeled cells return to the DNA synthetic zone to start synthesis for the next division, but a few labeled cells move beyond this zone and migrate into the primitive cerebral cortex (Fig. 4). These cells will become neurons.

To examine the migration path of newly formed neuroblasts from the neuroepithelial (matrix) layer toward their final position in the cortex, 12- to 17-day-old mouse embryos were labeled with tritiated thymidine and examined at various hours after treatment.[29] In all embryos sacrificed one to three hours after treatment, the label is almost exclusively limited to the neuroepithelial cell layer surrounding the lumen. During the following days, heavily labeled cells migrate from the neuroepithelial layer into the cortex. These cells, considered to be neuroblasts, pass through the cell layers formed on previous days. Cells labeled on day 14 of development reach the surface of the cortex just before birth (Fig. 5). On postnatal day 5, however, these heavily labeled cells are no longer located on the surface, but are separated from it by cells formed on days 15, 16, and 17 (Fig. 6). The latter cells have passed the layer formed on day 14

PLATE 2

5 Radioautograph of a coronal section through the cerebral hemisphere of an 18-day mouse embryo, 96 hours after treatment with tritiated thymidine (X100). The lumen of the ventricle (1), surrounded by the neuroepithelial zone (n.e.), is on the left of the figure. The heavily labeled cells, formed in the neuroepithelial layer on day 14, are located in the marked area along the surface of the cortex. Inset shows a number of heavily labeled neuroblasts as seen along the surface of the cortex under higher magnification (X540).

6 Radioautograph of a coronal section through the cerebral hemisphere of a 5-day postnatal mouse treated with tritiated thymidine on day 14 of gestation. The heavily labeled cells, formed on day 14, are now located in a rather sharply delineated zone (indicated by the dotted lines), and separated from the surface of the cortex by a zone of unlabeled and weakly labeled cells formed on days 15, 16, and 17. Inset shows some heavily labeled neuroblasts in the marked area under higher magnification (X1250).

Reprinted, by permission, from Langman, J. and Welch, G.W.: "Excess vitamin A and development of the cerebral cortex." J. Comp. Neur. 131: 15-26, 1967. (Courtesy of The Wistar Press.)

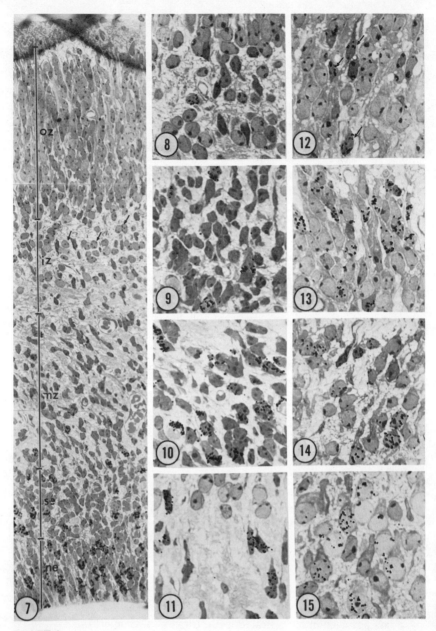

PLATE 3

7 Radioautograph of a section through the parietal cortex of a newborn hamster treated with tritiated thymidine one hour before sacrifice. The tissue was fixed in glutaraldehyde, embedded in araldite, cut at 1= and stained with toluidine blue. Note the radioactive cells in the neuroepithelial and subependymal layers. An occasional labeled cell was found in the

migratory zone. In the most superficial part of the inner cortical zone cells with a round nucleus, pale nucleoplasm, and one or two nucleoli adjacent to the nuclear membrane (arrows) are found. These cells, considered to be comparable to the round, dark-nucleated cells seen in the paraffin sections, are neuroblasts. The outer cortical zone contains cells with a spindle-shaped nucleus, as well as cells with an oval to round, pale-staining nucleus (X380).

8 Detail of the contact area between the inner and the outer cortical zones. In the lower part are visible cells with a round, pale-staining nucleus and in between them a few cells with a spindle-shaped nucleus. In the upper portion (outer cortical zone) are seen densely-packed cells characterized by a large, oval, pale nucleus. The labeled cell is related to a small blood vessel (X750).

9 Detail of the subependymal zone one hour after injection with tritiated thymidine. Note the great variation in nuclear shape. It is impossible to recognize any migrating neuroblasts (X750).

10 Detail of the subependymal zone 24 hours after injection with tritiated thymidine. The number of labeled cells has greatly increased in comparison with that in the previous figure. Some of the labeled cells are undoubtedly neuroblasts released by the neuroepithelium during the previous 24 hours. It is impossible, however, to distinguish migrating neuroblasts from the other labeled cells in the subependymal layer (X750).

11 Detail of the inner cortical zone 48 hours after treatment with tritiated thymidine. Note the labeled cells with a spindle-shaped nucleus and a cytoplasmic extension directed towards the periphery. The cells with the round, pale nucleus, comparable to the round, dark, nucleated cells of the paraffin sections, are not labeled (X750).

12 Detail of the superficial portion of the cortex 72 hours after labeling with tritiated thymidine. The first labeled cells with a spindle-shaped nucleus have now arrived at the surface of the cortex (arrows). The cells with an oval and round, pale nucleus are unlabeled (X750).

13 Detail of the superficial portion of the surface of the cortex 96 hours after treatment with tritiated thymidine. The labeled cells have lost their typical spindle shape as seen 24 hours earlier. The nucleus has become considerably paler and in some cells has become more oval (X750).

14 Detail of the surface of the cortex five days after labeling with tritiated thymidine. The labeled cells are now characterized by a round nucleus, pale nucleoplasm, and one or two distinct nucleoli close to the nuclear membrane.

15 Detail of the surface of the cortex nine days after labeling. The labeled cells are now characterized by a very large, pale nucleus and one or two distinct nucleoli close to the nuclear membrane. The cells are easily recognizable as neurons (X750).

Reprinted, by permission, from Shimada, M. and Langman, J.: "Cell proliferation, migration and differentiation in the cerebral cortex of the golden hamster." J. Comp. Neur. 139: 227-244, 1970. (Courtesy of The Wistar Press.)

and now occupy the most superficial position in the cortex. It is concluded that the neuroblasts of the neocortex are formed by the neuroepithelial cells surrounding the lumen. From there they migrate toward the periphery. The cells formed during the later stages of gestation bypass those formed at earlier days. The most superficial layer of the adult neocortex of the mouse is occupied by cells formed in the neuroepithelial layer on day 17 of development.

In the next series of experiments, the newborn hamster was used to examine the migration and differentiation of neuroblasts released by the neuroepithelial layer in more detail.[36] In the hamster, formation of neuroblasts continues until one or two days after birth. In Figure 7, a section is shown through the parietal cortex of a newborn hamster treated with tritiated thymidine one hour before sacrifice. Many neuroepithelial cells are labeled, although their number is not as large as during prenatal life. The subependymal layer, as well as the migratory zone, likewise contain a few labeled cells. The inner cortical zone with widely dispersed cells and the outer cortical zone with densely packed cells do not contain labeled cells, except an occasional one related to a blood vessel. In the inner cortical zone cells with a spindle-shaped nucleus and cells with a large, pale nucleus (neurons) can easily be recognized (Fig. 8). Twenty-four hours after treatment with tritiated thymidine the number of labeled neuroepithelial cells is about the same as at one hour after labeling. In the subependymal layer, however, the number is considerably larger (compare Figs. 9 and 10). Although, undoubtedly, a number of labeled cells in the subependymal layer are neuroblasts migrating from the neuroepithelium to the cortex, it is impossible to recognize these cells in the subependymal layer. The inner cortical zone, as well as the outer cortical zone, do not contain any labeled cells. Forty-eight hours after labeling, a number of labeled cells characterized by an elongated, spindle-shaped nucleus is seen in the deeper layers of the cortex (Fig. 11). None of the cells with an oval or round pale nucleus in the inner and outer cortical zones is labeled. At 72 hours after labeling the first labeled, spindle-shaped cells are observed at the surface of the cortex (Fig. 12). Four days after treatment most of the labeled cells at the surface of the cortex are either of the spindle-shaped type or characterized by an oval, light staining nucleus (Fig. 13). None of the neuroblasts or primitive neurons in the deeper layers of the cortex is labeled. By the fifth day the labeled cells at the surface of the cortex are now easily recognizable as small, round nucleated neuroblasts (Fig. 14). Nine days after treatment the labeled cells at the surface have the shape of large neurons (Fig. 15). From these observations it may be concluded that neuroblasts released by the neuroepithelial population migrate towards the surface of the cortex. The time needed for this migration is three to five days. As soon as the migratory cells reach the surface, the nucleus loses its spindle shape, becomes oval to round, while the nucleoplasm becomes pale. The cell then differentiates rapidly and obtains the form of a mature neuron.

In any consideration about growth and development of the central nervous system, three important areas will have to be taken into consideration: (1) proliferation including DNA synthesis; (2) migration from the neuroepithelial zone to the periphery; and (3) differentiation. Environmental factors may interfere with each of these three processes and, considering the abnormalities found in the human brain, it is not unlikely that if they interfere with proliferation, a neuronal deficit may result. If they interfere with migration, an ectopia of neuronal groups and layers may result; and if they interfere with cell differentiation, abnormal neurons may be found.

Many teratogenic factors, such as X-irradiation,[21,33] folic acid deficiency,[31,41] trypan blue,[15,20,43] excess vitamin A,[11,18] and dimethyl sulfoxide[16] cause exencephaly and anencephaly in mouse and rat embryos when administered to pregnant animals shortly before or during closure of the neural groove. When the same factors are given to pregnant animals much later in gestation after the neural groove has formed, no gross brain abnormalities are visible and the central nervous system seems to escape damage. A striking exception to this rule is formed by treatment with X-irradiation.[13,22,30] Exposure of rat embryos to 200r at later stages of development kills large numbers of differentiating and migrating neurons, while many proliferating cells around the ventricle degenerate. A somewhat similar example was found in some of our own previous work.[28] Excess vitamin A given to pregnant rats and mice during closure of the neural groove caused exencephaly and anencephaly in a high percentage of the newborn. When excess vitamin A was given sometime after closure of the neural tube, the production of neurons was lower than normal, and the migration and differentiation of existing neurons was abnormal.

Since considerable information is presently available about the day of birth of neurons in the neocortex,[5,6] hippocampus,[1,4] and other areas of the brain, as well as on migration and differentiation, the question was raised whether any environmental factors during prenatal life might interfere either with proliferation or with migration. To examine whether a short-term chemical insult during prenatal life would cause permanent damage to the brain in the form of a neuronal shortage or the presence of abnormal neurons, we selected for our most recent experiments 5-azacytidine, an analogue of cytidine.[26] This drug is known to have strong antileukemic properties[39] and to inhibit the growth of bacterial populations[10] and the root meristem of *Vicia faba*.[17] When injected into pregnant mice during the first half of gestation, the drug causes a high percentage of resorption of the embryos.[40] When given during later stages of development it was found to interfere with the mitotic activity of the neuroepithelial cells.[35] The chromosomes of the cells thicken and become arranged in irregular fashion. Whether this action is caused by interference of 5-azacytidine with RNA synthesis or indirectly with DNA synthesis is presently unknown. Figure 16 shows the cortex of a 15-day mouse fetus treated with

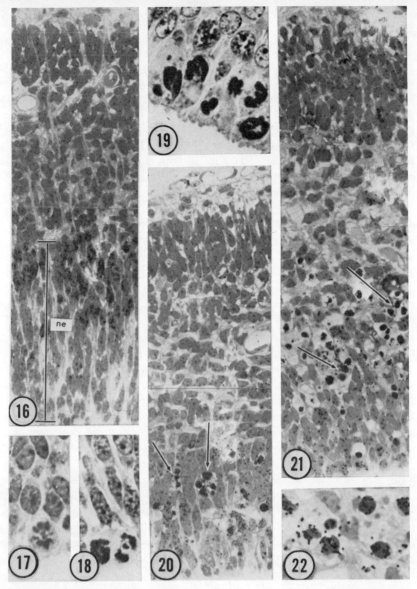

PLATE 4

16 Coronal section (1=) through parietal cortex of 15-day mouse fetus, treated with 5-azacytidine and one hour later with tritiated thymidine. The fetus was sacrificed 1 hour after the injection of tritiated thymidine. Pia is at the top and neuroepithelial layer (ne) at the bottom of the illustration. The labeled nuclei are in the outer zone of the neuroepithelial layer. No labeled cells are present in the migratory zone and cortical layers. The mitotic figures bordering the ventricular lumen are normal. Cresyl violet (X480).

17 Mitotic figure on the lumen of the ventricle of a 15-day fetus. Individual chromosomes can be clearly recognized (X1200).

azacytidine (4mg/kg) and tritiated thymidine one hour before sacrifice. Labeled nuclei are present in the outer zone of the neuroepithelial layer, but not in the migratory zone and in the cortical plate. The mitotic figures along the lumen are unlabeled and their chromosomal configurations are normal. The intensity of the label over the nuclei, as well as the localization of the labeled nuclei, was similar to that of the controls treated with tritiated thymidine only, indicating that 5-azacytidine does not prevent the incorporation of tritiated thymidine into DNA and does not block DNA synthesis.

Three to four hours after treatment, however, when the first labeled cells arrived at the lumen to divide, abnormal chromosomal configurations became visible. Initially, these abnormalities were relatively minor and consisted of abnormal chromosomal bridges and small clumps of chromosomal material (Fig. 18). A little later, however, the chromosomal abnormalities increased in severity. Since abnormal mitotic figures appeared about three to four hours after treatment, it seems likely that 5-azacytidine does not directly affect mitosis, but acts on the neuroepithelial cells during the DNA synthetic phase. In comparison to normal mitotic figures in which typical chromosomal patterns and individual

---

18 Mitotic figures along the lumen of the ventricle of a 15-day fetus, sacrificed four hours after treatment with 5-azacytidine. Note the abnormal chromosome configurations. Individual chromosomes cannot be distinguished and are seen clumped together forming comma and ring-shaped structures. Thin chromosomal bridges and isolated pieces of chromosomal material are also visible (X1200).

19 Mitotic figures along the lumen of the ventricle of a 15-day fetus, sacrificed 8 hours after treatment. Many abnormal mitotic cells have accumulated along the lumen, and the chromosomes are packed together forming ring and comma-shaped structures (X1200).

20 Coronal section (1=) through parietal cortex of 15-day fetus sacrificed 12 hours after treatment with 5-azacytidine and tritiated thymidine. The affected cells, most of which are labeled, are in the outer portion of the neuroepithelial layer. Some cells (arrow) contain three or more dark clumps of nuclear material (X480).

21 Coronal section (1=) through cortex of 16-day fetus, treated with 5-azacytidine and tritiated thymidine, and sacrificed 24 hours after treatment. Most of the affected cells are in the subependymal layer, but some have reached the migratory zone. They contain several dark clumps of nuclear material (arrows). The cytoplasm of the affected cells is pale (X480).

22 Detail of cells affected by azacytidine. Several clumps of labeled nuclear material are seen in a pale cytoplasm. Cell boundaries cannot be recognized (X1200).

Reprinted, by permission, from Langman, J. and Shimada, M.: "Cerebral cortex of the mouse after prenatal chemical insult." Amer. J. Anat. (in press), 1971. (Courtesy of The Wistar Press.)

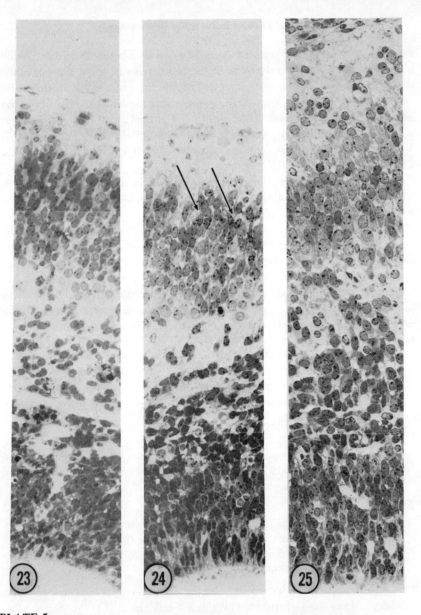

PLATE 5

23 Section (1=) through parietal cortex of the fetus treated with 5-azacytidine on day 15 of gestation and sacrificed 36 hours later. The pia is at the top and the neuroepithelial layer at the bottom of the illustration. Only a few cells with clumped nuclear material are present in the subependymal layer and migratory zone. Note the paucity of cells in the migratory zone (X480).

24 Section (1=) through parietal cortex of 17-day control fetus labeled with

chromosomes could be distinguished (Fig. 17), the chromosomes of the affected cells were clumped together, formed ring and comma shaped structures, and were attached to each other in many abnormal ways. These abnormal chromosomal configurations became more striking four to eight hours after treatment, when large numbers of dividing cells accumulated at the lumen (Fig. 19). During this time normal anaphases and telophases were absent. Despite the abnormal chromosomal patterns, the affected cells moved away from the lumen during the following 12 hours (Fig. 20). Twenty-four hours after treatment some of them had reached the migratory zone (Fig. 21). Many were extremely large, had a pale cytoplasm, and contained two to four darkly stained chromatin masses (Fig. 22).

Thirty-six hours after treatment most of the abnormal cells had disappeared and only a few clusters remained (Fig. 23). By this time the migratory zone seemed to contain fewer cells than the comparable layer in controls, but it was difficult to obtain accurate information since this layer is ill-defined. No abnormal cells could be found in any of the layers 48 hours after treatment.

Figure 24 shows the position of the labeled cells in the cortex of a 17-day fetus treated with tritiated thymidine 48 hours before sacrifice. Many labeled cells were noted in the cortical layers. Since DNA synthesis does not occur in the cells of the cortical plate (Fig. 16), the labeled cells must have migrated from the neuroepithelial zone toward the cortical plate. When similar animals treated with both 5-azacytidine and tritiated thymidine were investigated, labeled cells were not found in the cortical plate (Fig. 25), indicating that the cells affected by the 5-azacytidine must have died, thus causing a shortage of neuroblasts in the cortical plate. Surprisingly, when the cortex of newborn animals treated at day 15 of development was compared with that of untreated animals, it was difficult to detect any differences with morphological methods.

To investigate whether small doses of 5-azacytidine given at three successive days during pregnancy would cause a noticeable lack of neurons in the newborn cortex, pregnant mice were given 2 mg/kg azacytidine on days 13, 14,

---

tritiated thymidine 48 hours before sacrifice. Many labeled cells are present in the cortical layers (arrows) and migratory zone (X480).

25 Section (1=) through cortex of 17-day fetus treated with 5-azacytidine and tritiated thymidine 48 hours before sacrifice. None of the cells in the migratory zone and cortical layers is labeled (X480).

Reprinted, by permission, from Langman, J. and Shimada, M.: "Cerebral cortex of the mouse after prenatal chemical insult." Amer. J. Anat. (in press), 1971. (Courtesy of The Wistar Press.)

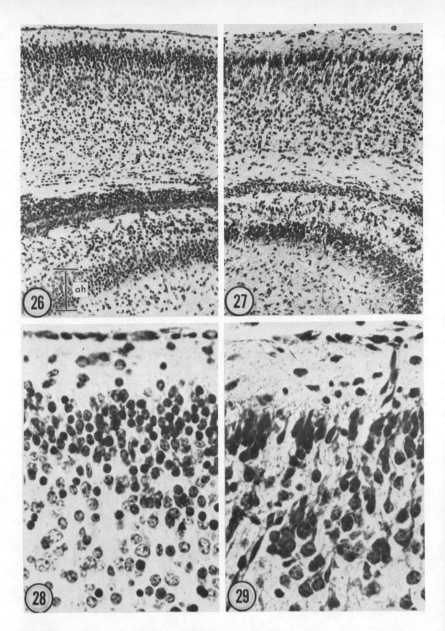

PLATE 6

26 Paraffin section (6=) through cortex and hippocampal region of newborn
control mouse. Note the neuroepithelial layers, the migratory zone (white
matter), and the various cell types in the cortical layers. The different
cortical layers, characteristic for the adult, cannot be distinguished since
most of the cells have not yet fully differentiated. The different layers of the
hippocampus, particularly the Ammon's horn (ah), are clearly recognizable
(X80).

and 15 of gestation. From Figure 27 it is evident that the brain of the treated newborn contained fewer cells than the control (Fig. 26). Similarly, the neuroepithelial layer and the layers of the hippocampal region contained fewer cells than the corresponding layers of the control (Figs. 26, 27). On higher magnification, it was noted that the cortex of the treated animals was characterized by many abnormal cells (Fig. 29). These cells, found mainly in the superficial layers of the cortex, were spindle-shaped and had a dark, round to oval nucleus. Corresponding cells in the controls had the appearance of normal differentiating neurons (Fig. 28). Similarly, in the hippocampal region many of the neurons in the Ammon's horn were disoriented, grossly abnormal, and degenerating (Fig. 31).

In addition, the cell number in the treated animals was considerably smaller than in the controls (Fig. 30). It is thus evident that repeated short-term treatments with small doses of 5-azacytidine cause a decrease in the total cell number in the cortex and that many surviving cells are abnormal in shape and possibly in function.

From the above experiments, it is evident that environmental factors can interfere with the production, migration, and differentiation of neurons in the central nervous system, even at late stages of development. Unfortunately, little is known about the manner by which environmental factors affect the central nervous system in human development. If malnutrition, as is presently suggested, interferes with the production of cells in the nervous system, we will first of all have to determine whether this effect is only on proliferating cells, or whether migration and differentiation are also affected. Once the mechanism of action is determined, we may be able to successfully attack the problem of malnutrition and brain development. Similarly, the question may be raised whether pollutants and drugs influence growth and differentiation of the human brain. Our

---

27 Similar section as in Figure 26 but from an animal treated with 2 mg/kg 5-azacytidine on days 13, 14 and 15 of gestation. The neuroepithelial and subependymal layers are thin and the number of cells in the migratory and cortical layers is much smaller than in the comparable layers of the control. Similarly the different layers of the hippocampal region contain fewer cells than those in the control (X80).

28 Enlargement of a portion of the superficial layers of the cortex shown in Figure 26. Note that the neuroblasts are in various stages of differentiation. Pia is at the top of the illustration (X500).

29 Enlargement of a portion of the superficial layers of the cortex as illustrated in Figure 27. The number of cells is considerably smaller than in the control, and many cells have a spindle-shaped nucleus, are darkly stained, and have an abnormal shape (X500).

Reprinted, by permission, from Langman, J. and Shimada, M.: "Cerebral cortex of the mouse after prenatal chemical insult." Amer. J. Anat. (in press), 1971. (Courtesy of The Wistar Press.)

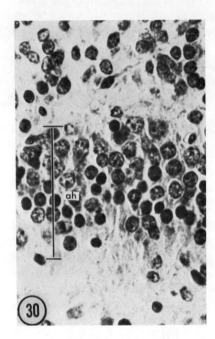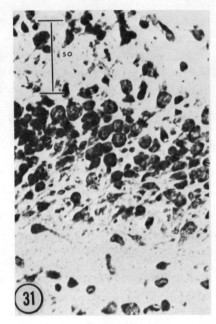

PLATE 7

30 Enlargement of a portion of the hippocampal region as shown in Figure 26.
Note the differentiating neuroblasts in the Ammon's horn (ah) (X1000).

31 Enlargement of a portion of the hippocampal region as shown in Figure 27.
Note the small number and abnormal form of the neuroblasts in the
Ammon's horn and stratum oriens (so) (X1000).

Reprinted, by permission, from Langman, J. and Shimada, M.: "Cerebral cortex
of the mouse after prenatal chemical insult." Amer. J. Anat. (in press), 1971.
(Courtesy of The Wistar Press.)

experiments clearly demonstrate that small chemical insults acting on the fetus
during its final stages of development may severely damage the brain. Whether
drugs and pollutants may exert a similar influence on the human brain remains a
question, but I believe that our experiments point out the way by which these
problems may be investigated.

(Editor's note: At this point, the meeting was opened to discussion. The
following are Dr. Langman's responses to questions.)

In present experiments, we have several groups of mice which have
survived the prenatal treatment for more than 90 days. To further investigate the

effect of the treatment, these mice are sacrificed at three-week intervals and stained with different neurochemical stains. The purpose of these experiments is to study which type of neuron has been most severely damaged, which type of neuron is absent, and whether or not the treatment has influenced the connections between neurons.

Behavioral and learning tests have not been performed to determine the damage caused to the neocortex and hippocampal region. Since our experiments show that it is possible to damage any population of cells of which the day of birth is known, it is evident that this method creates interesting possibilities to examine behavior and learning abilities in animals treated at specific days of development.

If newborn mice are treated at the day of birth or during one of the following days, serious clinical symptoms result. These animals are ataxic but manage to survive, possibly indicating that repair of damaged cells occurs. When in our previous experiments pregnant hamsters were injected with methylazoxymethanol on days 13-15 of gestation, most of the cells of the external granular layer of the cerebellum were destroyed at birth, although a few always survived.[37] By postnatal day 20, however, little difference in cytoarchitecture could be found between the cerebellum of the treated and the control animals, indicating that the surviving cells were able to repopulate the external granular layer, which in turn produced basket, stellate, and glia cells. A similar repair has been noted after X-irradiation. When early retina and associated eye structures in 13-15 day rat embryos and in 12½ day mouse embryos were exposed to 200r, virtually normal eyes developed, despite extensive damage to the tissues shortly after treatment.[23,34] In more recent experiments it was found that repair of the external granular layer is not restricted to damage suffered prenatally, but that exposure of the rat cerebellum to single and multiple doses of x-rays after birth also results in repopulation of the external granular layer.[37,38] In our own studies, in which repair of the external granular layer was studied after postnatal damage with 5-fluorodeoxyuridine and methylazoxymethanol, the cells of the proliferative population were able to compensate for cell losses suffered, but the repair did not result in a normal architecture of the cerebellum.[34,39] Hence, the cells of the external granular layer are apparently able to compensate for cell losses suffered during pre- and postnatal life, but the repair does not always result in a normal cerebellar architecture. The animals remained ataxic throughout the rest of their life.

Cell migration is, undoubtedly, one of the fundamental processes during development of the central nervous system. During the early stages of development, that is, during closure of the neural groove, the neuroepithelial cells form a pseudostratified epithelium. Even at later stages, the neuroepithelial cells are connected to the lumen with a long slender cytoplasmic process. At the lumen, the cells are connected to each other by terminal bars. Although the cell nucleus duplicates its DNA in the outer portion of the neuroepithelial layer, as soon as it is ready to divide, the nucleus migrates to the lumen and the cytoplasm contracts using the terminal bars as an anchor. Whether during this contraction a connection with the basement membrane is maintained is not known. As soon as the neuroepithelial cell has divided, one of the daughter cells moves to the outer layer of the neuroepithelial zone to begin DNA synthesis for the next generation, while the other daughter cell begins its migration to the periphery as a neuroblast.

As to the manner by which these cells migrate to their final position in the cortex, it has been stated that the neuroepithelial cells throughout development are characterized by two long cytoplasmic processes, one attached to the ventricular surface and the other to the pial surface.[7,8] During formation of the cortex, the peripheral processes never become dissociated from the surface of the cerebral cortex. The nuclei of these cells divide near the ventricular surface, but the cytoplasm does not divide. While one of the daughter nuclei remains near the ventricular surface, the other is thought to migrate towards the cortical surface within the cytoplasm of the peripheral process. After reaching the pial surface, the peripheral nucleus with scanty cytoplasm becomes independent. The neuroepithelial cell, however, maintains its connection to the pial surface. Although some Golgi-Cox preparations support this theory, considerable doubt remains as to the validity of this theory. The existence of long peripheral processes might be helpful in explaining the migration of neuroblasts from the neuroepithelial zone toward the cortex.

Presently, Dr. Butler, in our Department, is studying cellular migration in the cortex by means of electron microscopy.[9] In the past, this was impossible since we were unable to identify the migrating cell among the large number of differentiating neurons. By our labeling procedures, however, we are able to identify the migrating cells amidst the differentiating neurons. By examining the labeled cells two, three, and four days after treatment and studying their cell extensions and connections with other cells, maybe we can find long cytoplasmic extensions towards the periphery of the cortex. Although these experiments have not been finished, thus far we have not been able to identify a long process reaching towards the periphery. Similarly, we have not been able to identify any junctions with other cells. Hence, at present we do not have the slightest idea as to how cells migrate to their final position in the cortex.

I hope that in the future we can study these factors more in depth and that we will be able to discover which determinants affect the development of the central nervous system in the human fetus.

BIBLIOGRAPHY

1. Altman, J., "Autoradiographic and Histological Studies of Postnatal Neurogenesis. II. A Longitudinal Investigation of the Kinetics, Migration, and Transformation of Cells Incorporating Tritiated Thymidine in Infant Rats, with Special Reference to Postnatal Neurogenesis in Some Brain Regions," J. Comp. Neur., 128: 431-474 (1966).

2. Altman, J., "Postnatal Neurogenesis and the Problem of Neural Plasticity," *Developmental Neurobiology,* ed. by W.A. Himwich, Charles C. Thomas, Springfield, U.S.A., 197-237 (1970).

3. Altman, J., Anderson, W.J., Wright, K.A., "Early Effects of X-irradiation of the Cerebellum in Infant Rats: Decimation and Reconstitution of the External Granular Layer," Exp. Neur., 24: 196-216 (1969).

4. Angevine, J.B., Jr., "Time of Neuron Origin in the Hippocampal Region: An Autoradiographic Study in the Mouse," Exp. Neur. Suppl., 2: 1-70 (1965).

5. Angevine, J.D., Sidman, R.L., "Autoradiographic Study of Cell Migration During Histogenesis of Cerebral Cortex in the Mouse," Nature, 192: 766-768 (1961).

6. Berry, M., Eayrs, J.T., "Histogenesis of the Cerebral Cortex," Nature, 197: 984-985 (1963).

7. Berry, M., Rogers, A.W., "The Migration of Neuroblasts in the Developing Cerebral Cortex," J. Anat., 99: 691-709 (1965).

8. Berry, M., Rogers, A.W., "Histogenesis of Mammalian Cortex," *Evolution of the Forebrain,* ed. by R. Hassler, Stephen, H., Stuttgart, Georg Thieme Verlag, 197-205 (1967).

9. Butler, A.B., "The Migrating Neuroblast in Hamster Cortex: A Combined Autoradiographic and Electron Microscope Study" (in press).

10. Cihak, A., Sorm, F., "Biochemical Effects and Metabolic Transformations of 5-azacytidine in *Escherichia Coli,*" Coll. Czech. Chem. Commun., 30: 2091-2102 (1965).

11. Cohlan, S.Q., "Excessive Intake of Vitamin A as a Cause of Congenital Anomalies in the Rat," Science, 117: 535-536 (1953).

12. Cronkite, E.P., Fliedner, T.M., Bond, V.P., Rubine, J.R., Brecher, G., Quastler, H., "Dynamics of Hemopoietic Proliferation in Man and Mice Studied by H^3-thymidine Incorporation into DNA," Ann. N.Y. Acad. Sci., 79: 803-820 (1959).

13. Dekaban, A.S. "Differential Vulnerability to Irradiation of Various Cerebral Structures during Prenatal Development," *Radiation Biology of the Fetal and Juvenile Mammal,* Proc. of the Ninth Annual Hanford Biology Symposium. U.S. Atomic Energy Commission (1969).

14. Duncan, D., "Electron Microscopic Study of the Embryonic Neural Tube and Notochord," Tex. Rep. Biol. Med., 15: 367-377 (1957).

15. Ferm, V. H., "Teratogenic Effects of Trypan Blue on Hamster Embryos," J. Embryol. Exp. Morph., 6: 284-287 (1958).

16. Ferm, V.H., "Congenital Malformations Induced by Dimethyl Sulfoxide in the Golden Hamster," J. Embryol. Exp. Morph., 16: 49-54 (1966).

17. Fucik, V., Sormova, L., Sorm, F., "The Effect of 5-azacytidine on the Root Meristem of *Vicia Faba,*" Biologia Plantarum, 7: 58-64 (1965).

18. Giroud, A., Martinet, M., "Teratogenese par Hautes Doses de Vitamin A en Fonction des Stades du Developpement," Arch. d'Anat. Micr. Morph. Exp., 45: 77-98 (1965).

19. Giroud, A., Martinet, M., "Morphogenese de l'anencephalie," Arch. d'Anat. Micr. Morph. Exp., 46: 247-264 (1957).

20. Hamburgh, M., "The Embryology of Trypan Blue-induced Abnormalities in Mice," Anat. Rec., 119: 409-422 (1954).

21. Hicks, S.P., "Mechanism of Radiation Anencephaly, Anophthalmia, and Pituitary Anomalies, Repair in Mammalian Embryos," Arch. Path., 57: 363-378 (1954).

22. Hicks, S.P., D'Amato, C.J., "Effects of Ionizing Radiations on Mammalian Development," *Advances in Teratology,* London, Logos, 1: 195-250 (1966).

23. Hicks, S.P., D'Amato, D.J., Lowe, M.J., "The Development of the Mammalian Nervous System: I. Malformations of the Brain, Especially the

Cerebral Cortex, Induced in Rats by Radiation," J. Comp. Neur., 113: 435-469 (1959).

24. Langman, J., Guerrant, L., Freeman, B.G., "Behavior of Neuropithelial Cells during Closure of the Neural Tube," J. Comp. Neur., 127: 399-412 (1966).

25. Langman, J., Haden, C.C., "Formation and Migration of Neuroblasts in the Spinal Cord of the Chick Embryo," J. Comp. Neur., 138: 419-432 (1970).

26. Langman, J., Shimada, M., "Cerebral Cortex of the Mouse after Prenatal Chemical Insult," Am. J. Anat. (1971) (in press).

27. Langman, J., Sydnor, C.F., Haden, C.C., "A Radioautographic Study of the Origin of the Cellular Components in Chick Spinal Cord," Anat. Rec., 163: 215 (1969).

28. Langman, J., Welch, G., "Effect of Vitamin A on Development of the Central Nervous System," J. Comp. Neur., 128: 1-16 (1966).

29. Langman, J., Welch, G., "Excess Vitamin A and Development of the Cerebral Cortex," J. Comp. Neur., 131: 15-26 (1967).

30. Murakami, U., Hoshino, M., Kameyama, Y., "Mechanisms for the Differential Radiosensitivity of Immature Brain Tissue: Development of Hydrocephalus and Allied Conditions," *Radiation Biology of the Fetal and Juvenile Mammal,* Proc. of the Ninth Annual Hanford Biology Symposium, U.S. Atomic Energy Commission (1969).

31. Nelson, M.M., Asling, C.W., Evans, H.M., "Production of Multiple Congenital Abnormalities in Young by Maternal Pteroylglutamic Acid Deficiency during Gestation," J. Nutr., 48: 61-79 (1952).

32. Nygaard, D.F., Potter, R.L., "Effect of X-irradiation on DNA Metabolism in Various Tissues of the Rat," Radiation Res., 10: 462-476 (1959).

33. Rugh, R., Grupp, E., "X-irradiation Exencephaly," Am. J. Roent. Rad. Ther. Nuc. Med., 81: 1026-1052 (1959).

34. Rugh, R., Wolff, J., "Reparation of the Fetal Eye Following Radiation Insult," Arch. Ophthalmol., 54: 351-359 (1955).

35. Seifertova, M., Vesely, J., Sorm, F., "Effect of 5-azacytidine on Developing Mouse Embryo," Experientia, 24: 487-488 (1968).

36. Shimada, M., Langman, J., "Cell Proliferation, Migration, and Differentiation in the Cerebral Cortex of the Golden Hamster," J. Comp. Neur., 139: 227-244 (1970).

37. Shimada, M., Langman, J., "Rapir of the External Granular Layer of the Hamster Cerebellum after Prenatal and Postnatal Administration of Methylazoxymethanol." *Teratology,* 3: 119-134 (1970a).

38. Shimada, M., Langman, J., "Rapir of the External Granular Layer after Postnatal Treatment with 5-Fluorodeoxyuridine," Am. J. Anat., 129: 247-259 (1970).

39. Sorm, F., Vesely, J., "The Activity of a New Antimetabolite, 5-azacytidine, against Lymphoid Leukemia in AK Mice," Neoplasma, 11: 123-130 (1964).

40. Svata, M., Raska, K., Sorm, F., "Interruption of Pregnancy by 5-azacytidine," Experientia, 22: 53 (1966).

41. Tuchmann-Duplessis, H., Mercier-Parot, L., "Sur l'action Teratogene de l'acid X-methylfolique chez la Souris," C.R. Acad. Sc., Paris, 245: 1693-1695 (1957).

42. Tuchmann-Duplessis, H., Mercier-Parot, L., "A Propos de Malformations Produites par le Bleu Trypan," Biol. Med, Paris, 48: 238-251 (1959).

ACKNOWLEDGMENTS

These investigations were supported by research grant NB 06188 from the National Institute of Neurological Diseases and by grant R-200-66 from the United Cerebral Palsy Foundation. The author wishes to express his thanks to the following coworkers: Dr. G. Welch; Dr. C. Sydnor; Miss S. Haden and Dr. M. Shimada.

Genetic and Chemical Influences

Discussion

Orlando J. Miller

Not only is genetics the most important branch of medical science today, but it is also important in terms of the organization of scientific talent for effectively carrying out specific research projects.

To paraphrase Dr. Rosenberg, you pick an important problem in an area in which you have the greatest chance of accomplishing what you set out to do. At this particular time, I think his choice of a broad, multidisciplinary approach, including several basic sciences as well as research people at a medical school, is very important. Perhaps this is so in genetics more than in other areas, although after listening to the physiologists and considering how much all of us are dependent upon advances in computer technology, physics, and other basic sciences, it seems apparent that this is a general problem of all medical research. The few remarks I make will also emphasize how much each medical advance is based upon the prior development of new techniques and concepts which may come from scientists who are usually not identifiable as medical researchers at all. This is why I react so negatively to attempts to expand mission-oriented medical research at the expense of basic research, which is our life's blood.

I had planned to start with quite a different point. Dr. Rosenberg mentioned how important genetic disease is in the quantitative sense of numbers of people affected. We might rephrase this and ask how important genetic disease is as a cause of perinatal problems, e.g., picking specifically the problem of the low birth weight baby.

At this moment, even though the information is limited to perhaps 60 cases of the 5p deletion syndrome, it seems that about 1 in 500 premature births, of babies weighing less than 2500 g is due to the presence of a partial deletion of the short arm of the chromosome 5, that is, the Cri du Chat syndrome. The important feature here is not that this specific deletion is responsible for a large proportion of premature births. It is not, but it represents a category of disease where we can talk about cause and effect rather than simply speaking about correlations. This is one of the strengths of genetics, I think, that it offers us very helpful approaches to understanding the mechanisms underlying these problems. As Dr. Rosenberg has already pointed out, we do not yet know how chromosomal abnormalities produce abnormal phenotypes, but we at least know the nature of the question we must be able to answer in order to understand the problem.

If we consider the group of low birth weight babies who weigh less than 2,000 g, I would estimate that 1 in 500 is caused by a similar deletion involving the short arm of chromosome 4. There are a few other chromosomal abnormalities which are concentrated in the low birth weight of infants, but we can say little more about the role of deletions in causing these. This is primarily a technical problem, I think, in that the methods that have been available up to this point have been so very poor that we can only recognize a very small proportion of deletions which we have reason to suspect exist. So the real question is, are there new methods which might be used to extend our knowledge in this area?

There are, in fact, several new approaches that have been developed recently. Arrighi and Hsu have worked out one method which is based on molecular hybridization. In fact, they are using the person's own DNA molecules, denaturing the DNA of the chromosomes in standard metaphase preparations, allowing the rapidly reannealing DNA to renature and taking advantage of a property that most of us were not aware of, i.e., that many of the standard histological stains, such as Giemsa, have a greater affinity for double stranded DNA than they do for single stranded DNA. Fortunately, the rapidly reannealing DNA is not distributed along the chromosomes in a perfectly random fashion but tends to occupy specific locations. Consequently, you get identifiable patterns which can aid in identifying specific chromosomes. It is still uncertain whether this technique will be very useful, but approaches which take advantage of molecular properties of the chromosomes will ultimately be extremely important.

One of the people who worked with me a couple of years ago, Van

Freeman, used a similar approach. He made antibodies to the nucleoside bases of DNA, using a technique that was worked out by David Klein, Sam Beiser, and their associates at Columbia, tagged them with a fluorescent label, and studied their binding to human cells and chromosomes. The reason for doing this kind of study was that these antibodies have a specific affinity for single stranded DNA. What you get, in effect, is the complementary picture to that produced by the Arrighi and Hsu technique, which was unknown at the time of Van's studies.

I think that both of these methods have been overshadowed by one worked out by Caspersson over the last few years, a method which is based upon the ability of certain fluorescent chemicals to combine with DNA. The one that they found most useful was quinacrine mustard. What they found was that there are patterns of fluorescence along the chromosomes, reflecting consistent and characteristic differences in the binding of the agent to specific chromosomal regions.

Caspersson and his associates did most of their studies on plants. After a number of years, somebody encouraged them to look at human chromosomes. The result was the discovery that by this method you can identify virtually every chromosome in the human complement. The instrumentation that they used was so complex, I think it frightened most people. A number of people now—and I single out Roy Breg as one with, perhaps, the most experience and most convincing material—have found that very simple techniques, which are available in most clinical labs (as long as they have a fluorescence microscope), give surprisingly good results. You can use this simple technique to identify most of the chromosomes in the human complement, perhaps all of them. It is very easy to distinguish chromosome 21 from chromosome 22. I can state, on the basis of 10 cases we have studied with Roy Breg, that Down's syndrome is caused by 21 trisomy, that is, this condition is not produced by trisomy of the other chromosome in this group, number 22, but only by 21 trisomy.

You can also distinguish chromosomes 17 from 18 very clearly, and we have consistently found three chromosomes with one of these fluorescence patterns in cells from a patient with the 18-trisomy syndrome. Here, the previously used methods of autoradiographic analysis of terminal DNA replication were thought to be perfectly satisfactory in distinguishing between 17 and 18-trisomy. Autoradiographic studies of only one or two cases of 18 trisomy were ever reported, perhaps because the method was not all that effective.

The best part of the quinacrine-fluorescence technique is that you can identify individual chromosomes throughout the complement, e.g., 4, 5, the entire C-group of chromosomes 6 to 12, also the X and virtually all others. Furthermore, it is now possible with this technique to recognize inversions and other structural changes. We have shown that it is possible to distinguish translocation chromosomes from other chromosomes of the C-group that look much like them morphologically.

In short, I think we are moving to a higher level in terms of what we can accomplish with chromosome methodology. This will have implications all along the line. I think, for example, that all of the studies that have been carried out on the frequency of chromosome abnormality in abortions should be redone. The previous studies have defined fairly clearly the importance of numerical changes in chromosomes; trisomy, which occurs in something like 9 percent of all abortuses, triploidy, which occurs in about 4 percent, the 45,X or XO condition which occurs again in about 4 percent. There is very little information about structural changes, I suspect because of technical limitations of previous methods.

I think, with this fluorescence technique, it would be possible to find out what role structural changes play as a cause of abortion, and, perhaps, especially recurrent abortion. This may be important in assessing the mutagenic potential of the various environmental factors with which we are concerned, whether it is heavy metals or altitude or the host of mutagenic factors that we may know more or less about already.

One other point I want to mention is mapping the chromosomes. Here, too, I think, the development of new techniques is going to be extremely important. Already this fluorescent technique of chromosome identifications looks as though it is going to make it possible to recognize much greater numbers of chromosome markers which can be used with the classical types of linkage mapping, the kind that helped us to know that chromosome 1 carries the Duffy and zonular cataract loci. There is another approach which I suspect is going to be much more fruitful, and that is the technique of cell hybridization using Sendai or similar virus, or perhaps lysolecithin, to fuse the cells of two different species growing in tissue culture.

The species that has been most helpful so far in studying man is the mouse, because in man-mouse hybrid cells the human chromosomes tend to be thrown out, and you can force retention of a specific human chromosome by starting with a mouse cell line which is deficient in an enzyme that is necessary for survival in the presence of, say, aminopterin in the culture medium. This technique has already been used to map the thymidine kinase locus to human chromosome 17 or 18. Which of these two chromosomes is involved, undoubtedly will, I think, be determined by the fluorescent technique. The fact that we now know that a small E-group chromosome carries the thymidine kinase locus has come about through the use of cell culture, somatic cell genetic, and cell hybrid techniques.

There are other advantages to using cells in culture. It is possible to study a series of genetic markers that most of us have never thought about, for example, the susceptibility to polio virus. I think primates are the only animals that are susceptible to this virus, which will kill susceptible cells. Hybrid cells made by fusing human and murine cells, or human and hamster cells, are also susceptible to polio virus, but after enough human chromosomes are eliminated, as they are preferentially in these two hybrids, you may have a hybrid cell which is no longer susceptible to polio virus infection. This study was carried out by Howard

Green and his associates, who have tentatively assigned the locus for the presence of polio virus receptor onto a human acrocentric chromosome. This narrows the choice to five different chromosomes, but at least it shows the direction in which things are headed. I suspect that most of the assignments of specific human genes to chromosomes will be made using this kind of somatic cell genetic approach, using interspecific cell hybrids.

Perhaps I could make a few final remarks on a slightly different aspect of genetics. One of the chief advantages of the genetic methods of analysis is that they give us a lot more information about how sociological, infectious, heavy metal, or other environmental factors may operate in producing the effects which they have on individuals. There are various levels at which this can happen, all the way from their being mutagenic or teratogenic through a whole series of more complex interactions. The greater susceptibility of the sickle cell heterozygous carrier to anoxia would be one example. Another is genetically determined differential responsiveness to drugs. If you administer vitamin K to newborns, it is primarily the male with a G6PD variant who is going to be damaged by this. They are also at an increased risk to damage from a whole series of other drugs because of this enzyme deficiency.

What we are dealing with, in a sense, is the genetic basis for adaptation or maladaptation. Perhaps this would be a point to comment on an earlier comment made today: that the very rapid adaptation which occurred in the chick egg was an indication that the decisive factor was environmental rather than genetic. It is important to recognize that genetic adaptation can take place very quickly. In nature, each of us has to adapt, not simply to one environmental threat, but to all of the ones that we meet throughout our life up to the time of reproduction. For this reason, adaptation tends to be a very slow process. In a new situation, such as people going up to a very high altitude for the first time anyone in their family has done so for many generations, or an experimental situation where you are exposing animals to very low oxygen tensions, very large adaptive changes in gene frequency can take place in a single generation. I think perhaps an example would make this clear.

To use that classic genetic situation of a single locus with two alleles, big A and little a, and taking the gene frequencies for them as 90 percent ($p=.9$) and 10 percent ($1-p=.1=q$) respectively, there are three genotypes, the homozygous AA, the heterozygous Aa, and the homozygous aa. The frequencies of these three genotypes at equilibrium, usually they are not far off from this, are given by the Harry-Weinberg law: p^2AA:2pqAa:q^2aa, this is 81 percent, 18 percent, and 1 percent for AA, Aa, and aa respectively.

If we assume that anoxia will have a detrimental effect on the development of any individual with either the AA or Aa genotypes, then we could eliminate these from the next generation by subjecting chick eggs to anoxia. That would leave only 1 percent of the eggs, those of genotype aa. Since these would constitute the entire population, the gene frequency for the a allele will have gone from 10 percent to 100 percent in one generation.

Of course, there is now no genetic variation in this new population. If you put them back under the original conditions, growing the eggs at normal oxygen tension, you do not find the quick reversal that Dr. Metcalfe described. You can get around this by thinking about the way genes act, and assume that little a is a nonsense allele or something similar, so that the aa homozygote lacks the enzyme for which this is the structural locus. Heterozygotes usually show some variation in the amount of enzyme. If we were going to plot this graphically, with enzyme level along the X-axis, aa homozygotes would be concentrated at the left around zero enzyme. The normals would be far over to the right at high enzyme level, and the heterozygotes might show a normal distribution in the intermediate zone, which would overlap both the normal and abnormal ranges. The amount of overlap with the aa homozygote might be such that two of the 18 percent aa individuals would show almost zero enzyme. If so, then two-thirds of the survivors of the anoxia during embryogenesis would still have genetic variation at this locus despite the change in gene frequency, and the effect of selection would thus still be reversible.

You can work this out with two, three or more loci, in a very straightforward manner. The numbers are different, but the principle remains the same. Given the level of genetic diversity every human population appears to have, our genetic system, despite its stability, is not static. In fact, it provides an extremely rapid way for adapting to changes in our environment.

Developmental Genetics and Statistics

Discussion

James Miller

I should like to give some of my impressions of Dr. Rosenberg's presentation, and then comment on the topic "Developmental Genetics and Statistics" which links many of our common problems.

One of the big gaps in speaking about the matter of mechanics with which we must contend rests in that vast developmental void between observations made at the time of the birth of an individual and the molecular/biochemical considerations of early differentiation. Where have all the human embryologists gone?

We have heard a lot about the fetus during the past day and a half and now we are talking about molecular problems. What concerns me, simply stated, is "what happens to the organism between the time it implants and the time it gets to the stage of fetal development?" When I was a student, there were people, such as Bradley Patton, who were carrying out both active research and training people in the area of human embryology. Aside from sporadic reports, the literature in the field of human embryology is virtually nonexistent. It may be important to interest bright young people in the "embryology gap." Rather than being solely concerned with the problems of molecular differentiation, it would be more logical and of a higher priority if questions were asked of the sort that Hans Gruneberg and Sewell Wright have asked about gene action in experimental mammalian systems, particularly the mouse.[1,4] This involves the theoretically simple process of starting with a phenotype and then gradually working back through development, piecing in the picture, and eventually arriving at basic developmental processes. We do not seem to be able to do this, despite a tremendous volume of knowledge on gene-chromosomally-determined developmental errors in newborns and abortuses. For example, although we have a considerable body of information about the frequency and type of chromosomal aberrations in spontaneous abortions, we know virtually nothing of the nature of morphological errors in these specimens and the reasons for their death. We have some idea what the 45X phenotype is like, but we really do not know much about any others. What does the extra chromosome material or the rearranged chromosomal material do at the morphological level? The answer to this question is most important; eventually, it could have a significant application in preventive programs.

It is clear from the work of Caspersson and his colleagues in chromosome investigations that each of the chromosomes in the human complement can be clearly distinguished by its fluorescent staining pattern. These techniques have tremendous potential.

While I agree that genetic engineering, or whatever it is to be called, is exciting, I am somewhat concerned about it. My concern is not about the moral or ethical considerations, but about the implications of the fascination with this "panacea." Human beings are always captivated by solutions which may be just around the corner, "the big breakthrough," while ignoring those tools which are already at hand and which have great practical value. One of the most effective means of prevention of genetically-determined diseases at our disposal is genetic counseling. Most of the people in this country who need and require genetic counseling do not get it because they do not know it is available to them. Their physicians do not know enough to direct them to the genetic counselor. Personally, I find it somewhat distressing that we are talking about organ transplants, genetic engineering, and test tube babies, yet we do not seem to be able to provide citizens of this continent with the preventive services which are already proved and available.

Recently there has been increasing interest in societal problems of screening and monitoring for mutagenic and teratogenic effects of drugs, chemicals, and environmental pollutants in general. Despite all our technology and wealth of basic theory about how we should tackle the establishment of monitoring programs, we just do not know how to expedite them in a practical way. At the present time, our entire population could be exposed to a mutagen or teratogen which we would not be able to detect. If a workable detection system were established, how would we then go about looking for the one agent responsible among the hundreds to which the population is exposed daily?

Longitudinal studies are important. The value of having the ability to follow up individuals over long periods of time has been brought up in several ways at this meeting. Sir Dugald mentioned the possible impact of events during the depression on the reproductive capacity of women born during that period who are alive and reproducing now. This morning we talked about the value of following the reproductive pattern of women who themselves had certain congenital anomalies. Yesterday afternoon, there was concern about infections and the possibility that an initiating event may be separated by many years from the actual onset of a disease process or from a second event which then precipitated the disease state. The geneticist has worried about this in terms of following populations over long periods of time. Dr. Hellegers mentioned the value of linking the two forms of birth records—the official birth record and the physician's record. He implied that this could not be done, or at best would be difficult.

I should like to suggest that the tools for carrying out such longitudinal studies are available to us in the form of record linkage technology. Newcombe in Chalk River, Ontario, has used the Province of British Columbia's vital records to demonstrate the feasibility of linking many records. He has linked birth records, physician's notice of birth records, death records, stillbirth records, and records from a handicapped children's registry.[2] He has computerized a fairly complete picture of reproductive events over the past 20 years in the Province of British Columbia. Newcombe is primarily concerned with this linkage technology from a genetic point of view. These techniques are of significance for many problems in human biology, some of which we are concerned with at this meeting.[3] Dr. Dornbusch said it would be the notable physician who was able to follow individual patients over many years and keep meaningful records of significant events. No physician can do it. The problem is beyond one man. It is only by using computer technology over a long period of time that we will be in a position to analyze many of the problems with which we are confronted.

There is one aspect about the potential use of such techniques that disturbs many people. This concerns the problem of the maintenance of confidentiality of the volumes of information contained in such linkage systems. There is tremendous concern in this country and elsewhere about data banks in general. There has to be concern about protecting the confidentiality of the personal medical and sociological information which is stored in systems such as those developed by Newcombe. Many of the questions for which we are desperately seeking answers can only be resolved by such systems. We will be forced to make some major decisions as to how we are going to use this machine technology to answer questions which are of great relevance to the health status of the citizens of an industrialized society. It must be recognized in establishing and maintaining these systems that the confidentiality of the information available must be scrupulously respected. Although the final solution to this dilemma will not be easy, I firmly believe it is imperative that it be achieved as quickly as possible.

BIBLIOGRAPHY

1. Gruneberg, *The Pathology of Development,* New York, Wiley, 1963.

2. Newcombe, H.B., Rhynas, P.O.W., "Family Linkage of Population Records," *The Use of Vital and Health Statistics for Genetic and Radiation Studies,* New York, United Nations, 135-153 (1962).

3. *Record Linkage in Medicine,* ed. by E.D. Acheson, Edinburgh, Livingston, 1968.

4. Wright, S., "Summary of Patterns of Mammalian Gene Action," J. Natl. Can. Inst. 15: 837-851 (1954).

General Discussion

One of the problems with genetics and genetic counseling pointed out by Dr. Dancis was that the confidentiality of the material obtained from the patient must be preserved. The question is what to do when the confidentiality of the material is contrary to the best interest of society. In general, the group agreed that this was a problem that would best be handled on an individual basis. Consanguinity is one of the problems constantly encountered in genetics, and Dr. James Miller indicated that attitudes toward consanguinious marriages has varied widely in different cultures. However, with our knowledge of genetics it would be important to prevent consanguinious marriages when there is a greater chance for genetic abnormalities.

Dr. Behrman asked why genetic counseling need be done by a physician. He thought the utilization of genetic data could be done by other medical personnel and that the physician could use the genetic counseling session as an aid for guidance of his patients. Dr. Rosenberg brought out that there are many kinds of genetic counseling: there is a type of genetic counseling which needs a professional geneticist and another which requires the expertise of a physician. Physicians must be better trained in genetics so that they can perform adequately in the counseling of individuals. The problems with genetic counseling are: what does the patient learn from the counseling and once having been counseled, will the patient take the advice of the counsellor in the conduct of his life? Dr. Gordon reiterated many of the comments by Dr. Rosenberg and further emphasized that in genetic counseling there are personal ethical concepts that may be interfered with by the counseling. He further said that there has been a great deal of help, in terms of genetic disease, by liberalization of abortion laws in a variety of states.

Behrman posed a rather provocative question to the geneticists by asking what kinds of research problems are most important to the geneticist. After some discussion, this was replied to, reluctantly, by the group of geneticists. Rosenberg thought it was essential to study ways by which cells can be grown more effectively and rapidly in tissue culture. He thought that if we could speed up the process of growing cells, then antenatal diagnosis would be enhanced enormously. He also indicated that an understanding of the genetics of development is probably the most important problem facing the human geneticist at present. Dr. O. J. Miller stated that he and other human geneticists in the audience could not be regarded as spokesmen for the field. Genetics is one of the many basic sciences contributing to the health of man. He also thought that mapping of chromosomes is an extremely important problem to be solved. He used as an example the recent report on myotonic dystrophy which is caused by a mutant gene linked to the secretory locus. The secretory locus can be recognized in cells of the amniotic fluid and, consequently, the potential for myotonic dystrophy can then be determined *in utero*. Another area of extreme importance to study is linkage. This information would be helpful in delineating functional groupings of genes. One example is that the entire chromosome could be considered to be a genetic unit. The beauty of linkage studies is to show relationships between organisms which could indicate a common mechanism for control of specific genetic functions. Rosenberg said that it would be very important if the genetic control for the hemoglobins could be discovered, since the information could be applied to sickle cell anemia. Dr. James Miller indicated that one of the ways to determine genetic disease in a country is to conduct epidemiological studies for estimation of the occurrence of genetic disease. Dr. Segal stated that a number of hospitals are destroying old records and that possibly some mechanism for storage of records should be established. Apparently, the United Kingdom has been contemplating the establishment of community banks for long-term storage. Dr. Ransome-Kuti indicated that in Nigeria they permit patients to keep their own records which they do very well. Dr. Barnett questioned the association of 21 trisomy with Down's syndrome. Dr. O. J. Miller indicated that this particular karyotype has not been encountered with any other phenotype. In regard to Dr. Langman's talk, Dr. Sereni brought up the question as to the mechanism responsible for migration of cells in the cerebellum of the rat during development. Dr. Langman said that he wished he knew, but that it might be possible to think of chemotaxis as a mechanism.

This area certainly requires further research. Dr. James Miller queried Dr. Langman on his use of random or inbred strains of mice. Dr. Langman indicated that his work was conducted with mice of an inbred strain. Similar experiments have been done with rats and hamsters. There are species differences. In the mouse and the rat, the formation of neurons for the neocortex is complete before birth. In the hamster, this process continues for approximately two days after birth. Dr. Gordon asked Dr. Langman whether there were effects of protein malnutrition which would affect one strain and not another. He pointed out that it would be very difficult to extrapolate from a pure strain to the heterozygousity of the human. Langman indicated that he was aware of the problem, but, nonetheless, there are many environmental factors which influence the mouse fetus late in pregnancy that can cause abnormalities in production and differentiation of neurons.

Aspects of International Perinatal Research

Introduction

Norman Kretchmer

Although scientific information is readily disseminated throughout the world, it is used in different ways, depending upon the local needs, conditions, and economic development.

We were fortunate that Professors Alexander Minkowski, Ettore Rossi, and Fabio Sereni were in the United States at the time of this conference, and that they were willing to participate in the proceedings. Professor Ransome-Kuti was urged to attend so that we could have the benefit of his vast medical and scientific experience in West Africa.

These scholars represent only two areas of the world, but they bring essential information which defines their problems as well as the roles of various nations.

Some of the problems they will discuss are unique to their own areas and some are shared by all. Perinatal biology knows no boundaries.

Panel

O. Ransome-Kuti

I believe that it is important to indicate some aspects of pediatrics with which you may not be familiar. Usually, when a paper is sent to an American journal for publication by my countrymen, we receive this reply: "We are very sorry we cannot print your paper. It has been 20 or 30 years since we observed the condition that you describe in this country." Consequently, I will use the present opportunity to relate the perinatal problems one encounters in Nigeria and the types of research in progress.

Nigeria is a continually developing country and, as a result, few complete statistics are available. Thus, without solid vital statistics, it is difficult to define the problems clearly and to undertake an appropriate course of action.

A very high infant and child mortality rate exists in Nigeria, and only conjectures can be offered as to why children live or die. However, we know some of our priorities, and one of them is to collect accurate statistics.

There is little attempt to collect vital statistics in the North. In Katsina, the Department Secretary of the Administration, Ministry of Health, has been attempting to collect data on stillbirths and deaths of the newborn by questioning village heads. Every family must report to the village head the death of any child upon delivery. He, in turn, must relate this information in written form to the Administrative Center. We discovered that the collector of statistics was confused as to what data he was supposed to assemble. He had been gathering information on any type of death, for example, abortions. Thus, there was some difficulty with the interpretation of the results.

The only valid statistics available are hospital statistics. These data are unreliable in many cases because their collection is left in the hands of nurses and paramedical people. In the teaching hospitals the cases are selective, and the data are not representative of perinatal mortality in the country. We conjecture that our perinatal mortality (less than 24 hours) would be about 30 per 1,000 live births. Lagos has a maternity hospital in which there are 24,000 births a year and 70 to 80 babies born each day. The mothers spend from 6 to 12 hours in the hospital. Follow-up data on the babies are not maintained, so mortality statistics are not known.

There are only 14 beds for neonates in Lagos, all of which are at University College Hospital. A facility exists in the maternity hospital for both well and sick newborns, but it does not function as a modern neonatal unit. A ward for neonates is now being opened with an additional 30 beds in University College Hospital. With this new facility there is the possibility of caring for many of the neonatal problems in Lagos. There are 25 neonatal beds in University College Hospital in Ibadan. The mission hospitals in Ilesha, which are very good units, may have more beds. There is no functioning neonatal unit in the whole of the Northern region, an area which occupies more than half of the country. It is estimated that only 3 percent of our mothers obtain general and perinatal care in Nigeria. These are some of the problems with which we must cope.

The most common problem and cause of death is prematurity, which is due perhaps to the faulty antenatal care. This problem may result from cultural mores involved in care of our mothers, since many taboos exist regarding what mothers should and should not eat. Twinning is very common. The Yoruba are famous for bearing twins and triplets. West Africa probably has the highest twinning rate in the world, 1 in 20, as compared to the figures for the Western World of 1 in 80. These are just a few reasons for the high rate of prematurity.

Many infants die because of the poor facilities available for treatment. When a premature infant is admitted to a general ward, infection and death are imminent. Asphyxia is commonly quoted as a high cause of death in the records of our maternity hospital. This problem results from too few pediatricians and nurses having knowledge of simple methods of resuscitation. Toxemia is very common and serves as a real cause for prematurity.

There are many cases of tetanus, although it is a preventable disease and should not occur. In Lagos, for the first time in Nigeria, general steps are being taken to immunize mothers against tetanus. Upon visiting a maternity hospital, I ventured to query, "Why don't you immunize the mothers against tetanus?"

they responded, "The mothers are delivered in this hospital in very hygienic conditions, and their babies do not contract tetanus. Women who should be immunized against tetanus are those who are unable to deliver in the maternity hospital." Within two to three months I saw 25 infants who had been born in that maternity hospital, and who were discharged within six hours and brought to University College Hospital with neonatal tetanus. I sent their names and addresses back to the maternity hospital. As a result, the Hospital began to immunize the mothers against tetanus. Other causes of tetanus are umbilical sepsis, the practice of female and male circumcision during the first week of life by native doctors, tribal marks on the face, and the practice of delivering their children on the bare floor.

Once, in Ibadan, we visited homes of those mothers whose babies had tetanus. All samples taken from the floor at random had tetanus spores in the culture. It is a practice of our people to deliver their babies on the floor, and yet many people see no reason for the prevalence of tetanus. It is interesting that tetanus in the newborn is our number-one problem met on an emergency-room basis.

Another problem, as a result of Rh incompatibility, is jaundice in the newborn. This disease has been a personal source of interest for a long time. This year, with the help of Dr. N. Kretchmer, we have begun to tackle the problem scientifically. Some studies have indicated jaundice among normal male babies, because of our interest in G6PD deficiency. Babies who left the hospital never had bilirubins which rose above 10 mg per 100 ml. Every infant with a total serum bilirubin above 10 mg per 100 ml was investigated for a cause of jaundice.

The most common cause of jaundice is G6PD deficiency, which, we think, is the major reason for neonatal jaundice. Infants are also tested for Rh incompatibility, ABO incompatibility, Coombs' test, blood culture, and liver function.

Jaundice in association with G6PD deficiency must result from something the mothers do to their babies at home. Perhaps a drug is used or perhaps the children's clothes are put into naphthalene. The exogenous factors causing jaundice in these babies is unknown.

G6PD deficiency, plus infection, is also prevalent. The infection may trigger hemolysis.

Some newborns are G6PD deficient as well as ABO incompatible. The Coombs' test in most of these children is negative. Those with ABO incompatibility constitute another group with jaundice.

In 18 percent of the outpatient group with jaundice, there is no known cause for the jaundice. It is striking that jaundice is the second most common cause of death of the newborn in Nigeria, and the most common cause of cerebral palsy. In cord blood taken from the infants born in the North, G6PD deficiency is encountered in the same frequency as in the West, but jaundice is infrequent in the North. This is a question which deserves a response.

Tetanus in the newborn is also uncommon in the North. Interestingly, the largest population of goats, cows, donkeys, and camels is concentrated in the North, and the people virtually live with their animals. During this close habitation with the animals, it is feasible that the mothers acquire small doses of tetanus toxins and have become immunized, and thus, are able to pass the antibodies on to their babies.

In the inpatient group of the newborn babies, those who are born and cared for in the neonatal unit in the hospital, the most common cause of jaundice is ABO incompatibility.

The second most common cause of jaundice is G6PD deficiency. Approximately 28 percent are ABO incompatibility, whereas approximately 21 percent are G6PD deficiency. Approximately 8 percent are G6PD deficiency plus ABO incompatibility. In this group of patients, there is a preponderance of males over females.

With approximately 30-35 percent of the jaundice cases, there was no cause. The bilirubins in these cases is usually greater than 10 mg per 100 ml and some of these babies need to have their blood exchanged.

A common cause of death or disease among the newborns is infection. In the outpatient group, bronchopneumonia, umbilical sepsis, conjunctivitis, pemfigus, neonatorum, and staphlacoccus infection are common causes. There are also some cases of toxoplasmosis and rubella syndrome.

Rubella syndrome deserves some examination. There have been only four or five cases in the last seven years in Lagos. A study of rubella antibodies showed that 98 percent of all girls had had rubella before they entered the University. Therefore, the majority of our mothers have had rubella before giving birth. How these four or five babies escaped and how their mothers escaped getting rubella before they came to childbirth is unknown.

A visual study of 24,000 births in the Maternity Hospital during one year showed that the frequency of congenital malformation in Nigeria is the same as has been reported in the United States and in Great Britain. Polydactylia is the most frequent of visible malformations.

In summary, the factors responsible for the high perinatal mortality and morbidity in Nigeria are the following: (1) lack of medical facilities, (2) lack of medical personnel, and (3) socioeconomic factors.

In regard to facilities, the medical services must be organized. Past efforts have been haphazard and disjointed. An organization must be formed with the implicit goal of assuring every pregnant woman antenatal care. Domiciliary care must be expanded so that someone can be sent into each home to check on the progress of each pregnant woman.

Rural centers should be established, staffed by auxiliary personnel trained in the common care of pregnant women, the delivering of babies, and they should be taught to recognize any possible danger signs in the mother and baby. As a result, people could be referred from these rural centers to suburban health centers where better facilities exist.

A committee has been established to organize such a health service system in Nigeria. The mother's whereabouts are inconsequential, because she will be assured treatment in the rural health centers, suburban health centers, and ultimately shifted into a hospital equipped with trained auxiliary personnel. Until our socioeconomic conditions improve, we will not be able to effect a meaningful decrease in our mortality rate.

Health education is very important and research must be carried out. How does the information reach the mother? In every clinic in Nigeria, every doctor and every midwife is practicing health education. The mothers are told what we think is best for them, but our efforts to reduce the mortality rate have been in vain.

Discussion of malnutrition with mothers has led to no overt advances. Mothers had been told what the children should eat. When they come to the clinic, we ask, "What should you give your child?" She answers, "Meat, fish, eggs and vegetables." We then ask, "What do you give your child?" "I give him pap." "And what else?" "Just pap." The mother is aware of what her child needs but ignores our pleas. We are in the process of collecting data on the beliefs of our people in regard to the causes of various diseases in the country, such as anemia, tetanus, and pneumonia. Until we know more about their actual beliefs and their practices in relation to these diseases, our health education programs cannot be successful.

In consideration of pollution, many mothers sit in a closed room in front of a wood fire throughout their pregnancy. They inhale a high percent of carbon monoxide from ovulation to parturition. The epidemiology of bronchial pneumonia has been studied. An individual from rural health visited the home of every bronchial pneumonia patient and took gas samples. We found that the majority of these children came from homes in which the mother strapped the child to her back and sat in a smoke infested room. The child is forced to stay in that position and inhales the very dangerous gases containing sulfides and benzene compounds while the mother cooks. Consequently, the child enters the hospital with bronchitis and bronchopneumonia.

Lactose intolerance and breast-feeding is a very interesting problem. A study of this kind has been conducted before, but there was no follow-up. We found that more than 90 percent of the people of my tribe, including myself, are lactose-intolerant. What bearing would this observation have on the feeding of milk to children? What bearing would it have on convulsions? Many of our children have convulsions. Some are hypoglycemic and have convulsions. Is it because they are not absorbing any glucose or have no glycogen stores?

Only through research and education can we effectively advance our ability to reduce the number of perinatal problems in Nigeria.

Alexander Minkowski

It is extremely important to be able to determine the eventual neurological prognosis for the premature infant in an intensive care nursery. We have been interested for some time in the early development of the central nervous system. As a result of this interest, we have studied the basic problems connected with intrauterine growth retardation. We are all interested in the exact relationships between malnutrition occurring pre- and postnatally and the way the baby is fed in relation to the further development of the brain.

The development of the brain is affected by a number of phenomena, i.e., hypoxia, acidosis, cold, etc. We still have to know the cerebral limits of tolerance to environmental factors and what adjustments the brain makes to particular situations. The central nervous system pursues its own growth, regardless of the direction of general growth. There may, however, be nonrecognized lesions in the central nervous system. In fact, if you examine an infant weighing 1 kilo, he will have almost the same degree of maturation of the brain as the baby who weighs 3 kilos.

Study of early development has value as a possibility for assessing gestational age. In some instances, an EEG provides a rather accurate way of assessment. A very interesting phenomena occurs in the EEG at 37 weeks of gestation. There is synergy between two hemispheres, which may mean that each hemisphere is acting in an independent fashion. This finding in the EEG is age-dependent and is the same regardless of whether the child weighs 1 kilo or 3 kilos. This conclusion has been found to be correct in 86 out of the 96 patients evaluated.

The problem of intrauterine growth retardation illustrates some interesting developments in our field of research. Data obtained from human beings and animals shows a striking discrepancy of involvement between different organs during intrauterine growth retardation. Despite the fact that the rat is not an ideal animal for the study of intrauterine growth, it serves as a good model. By ligation of one uterine artery, at the 17th day of gestation, "small-for-dates" animals can be produced on one side of the uterus and the other horn can be used as a control. Retardation greater than 15 percent in body reduction is considered to be significant.

Twelve days after birth, the animals are still small and they do not catch up. We must differentiate between those that catch up quickly, those that catch up normally, and those that never catch up. By comparing the weight of organs in intrauterine growth retardation, there is a significant reduction of the liver weight, but there is relatively no reduction in the weight of the brain.

The same findings are encountered in the human. On the average, in rats, there is approximately 35 percent reduction in total body weight. The reduction of liver weight is considerably higher, 60 percent. The liver is much more affected than total body weight, but the brain is very slightly reduced in size. Many enzymatic studies have been accomplished in our laboratory, i.e., glucose 6-phosphatase, lactase dehydrogenase, fructose diphosphatase, aspartate-amino transferase. There were no differences between the control animals and those with growth retardation. There is no catch up of total body weight or the weight of the liver by the 20th day.

If one examines the cerebral hemispheres, there are no differences in the total DNA content in the cerebrum from day 1 to day 20. The total DNA is exactly the same in the control and in the rats that are small-for-dates. Cell size can be grossly estimated from the ratio of protein to DNA. Except for the first few days, there is no major difference in cell size. The major index indicates that there is an enormous reduction of cells in the liver and almost no reduction of the number of cells in the brain. If incorporation of radioactive thymidine is measured into the liver and the brain of the retarded rats, it is noted that the radioactivity in the liver is considerably diminished, while there is no change in the cerebral hemispheres.

These kinds of experiments can serve as a basis for the study of the relationship between brain development and malnutrition. In addition, there are other fruitful areas to be pursued. For example, pharmacologic studies are very important. We recently discovered a number of cross-infections in the nursery. One source of contamination comes from the products that we use in the care of the baby, such as drugs, ointments, and solutions delivered either by the pharmacy or by companies. We are studying this problem in conjunction with the bacteriologists at the Pasteur Institute.

Klebsiellae, which are highly pathogenic organisms, are sometimes found in the products used in the unit. We asked the manufacturer to prepare a sterile preparation of mycostatin, which cost about ten times more than usual. I would propose this possibility as a serious potentiality for contamination in the nurseries. Finally, something that relates to what was said yesterday about pollution. It concerns the action of defoliating products of herbicides. A report from the NIH has shown that at certain doses, the products called 2,3,5-T and 2,4-D are 100 percent teratogenic to the animal. These data cannot be extrapolated to the human, but they should be recognized as pertinent observations. In California, Vietnam, and other places where insecticides are used, a survey should be made to determine whether there is an increase in the frequency of congenital malformations. This problem should be studied and is certainly important in our field. We know that it is extremely difficult to obtain valid epidemiologic data on such a subject. (Editor's Note: Dr. Minkowski discussed, off the official record, the indiscriminate use of herbicides and antifoliates in Vietnam.)

Another interesting avenue for investigation is the study of blood and oxygen consumption of the brain. We have made some determinations of cerebral blood flow, obtaining our specimens from indwelling catheters in the heart, the carotid artery, or jugular vein. We are, however, reluctant to generalize at this time. Another one of the major problems for study is the effect of separation from the mother and its role in the later development of these infants.

Delivery of health care is generally somewhat a socio-political problem. In certain countries, they utilize methods to insure that every pregnant woman will receive proper care. In the field of preventive medicine, countries like Red China employ special ways of surveying the pregnant woman. Health surveys are compulsory over the entire country. For instance, each pregnant woman has her blood pressure taken every week as well as other very simple determinations. They claim that toxemias have disappeared in China with the use of these measures.

I have discussed some of the areas of study going on in my laboratory and also have highlighted some important projects that should be pursued further.

Ettore Rossi

My purpose, together with that of Sir Dugald, Minkowski, and Sereni, is to discuss, very briefly, some problems concerning perinatology in Europe.

If the perinatal period is defined as the time span between the 28th week of gestation and the first postnatal week, then the perinatal mortality in Europe dropped sharply between 1956 and 1966. The differences in the various countries are associated with socioeconomic and medical social factors.

The perinatal mortality in Switzerland decreases less than the infant mortality. Not only do environmental factors play a role, but so do genetic and constitutional factors. For this reason, since 1968, there has existed a European Society for Perinatology. Two congresses of this Society have been held: one in 1968 in Berlin with more than 1,000 people in attendance, and another in 1970 in London. The next will be held in 1972 in Lausanne.

Statistical evaluation is submitted to careful criticism, indicating that one of our priorities in perinatology is to view the problem on a statistical basis. There are teams in Finland, Sweden, and Switzerland working to define various path-physiological states in causation of perinatal mortality, so as to have a critical statistical evaluation of the problem.

The perinatal mortality rate is generally between 19 and 43.6 per 1,000 live births.

There are many countries so dissimilar that it is difficult to make a comparison. For instance, in Holland, 80 percent of the children are born in the home. There is no opportunity for comparison. In the Northern European countries, there are more laboratories, and they can follow the babies easier than in Southern Europe. Thus, the interpretation and comparison of the different statistics is very difficult.

Low birth weight is a problem which deserves careful consideration. There is an increase in the percent of low birth-weight infants being born. There is an increase in the perinatal mortality in different countries in Europe. In Hungary, one finds the highest percent of low birth-weight children and the highest infant mortality rate. England has a higher perinatal than fetal mortality rate.

The major cardiorespiratory research centers are in Sweden and in England: Lind and Kalberg in Sweden, and Strang and Tizard in England. In Switzerland, Prod'hom is working on these questions and now is classifying the different forms of respiratory distress syndrome. In Italy, Bucci is working in a similar area.

The perinatologists in Goteborg until recently studied pulmonary and respiratory questions; now they are studying cardiovascular and neurological physiology. The same is true of Prechtl in Groningen, Schulte in Gottingen, and Minkowski in Paris. In Switzerland, Rabinowitz is compiling an atlas describing changes of the central nervous system in the low birth-weight newborn. A group in my department is studying the psychological development of the infant.

There are a number of groups studying metabolic problems. Zetterstrom is working on carbohydrate and neonatal hypoglycemia; also, there is Milner in Manchester, Meyer in Louvain, Grasso and Sereni in Italy, Pederson in Denmark, and Zurbrugg in Berne. In the field of endocrinology are: Malvaux in Belgium, Anderson in Denmark, Teller in Germany, Jost in France, and de Olin in Sweden. Steroid metabolism is studied by Rappoport in France, Visser in Holland, Diczfalusy in Sweden, and in our department.

We are trying to found a new organization dealing with perinatal problems. The purpose is to study groups of 500,000 people in distinguishable countries and to attempt to have for these 500,000 a doctrine designing the care of the mother and the child.

Fabio Sereni

I will incorporate some data concerning the future of research in perinatology in Western Europe, which I have gathered as general secretary of the European Society for Pediatric Research. The European Society of Pediatric Research was founded three years ago, and presently has about 150 members representing many countries from Eastern and Western Europe. There is a very high representation from the Northern countries: England, France, West Germany, Holland, and Denmark. A low representation of research workers come from lower income countries: Italy, Spain, Portugal, and the Eastern European countries.

Pediatric research is not so advanced in many countries in Europe but varies from time to time and from country to country. The lack of good medical schools and research tradition is a problem in Italy, as well as for many other countries.

The most crucial problem resulting from the reduction of funds for basic research in the U.S.A., when this is considered from the point of view of a European pediatrician, is the question of the future of the medical school and the training of postgraduate students in research in those countries where at present there is no high standard of research.

There have been approximately 50 applications for active membership in the European Society of Pediatric Research in the past two years. Eighteen of the applicants were interested in problems of the fetus or of the newborn. Among these, 5 were interested in clinical problems; 9 in the physiology of the perinatal period of life, and the other 4 in developmental pharmacology. We have neither an embryologist nor a teratologist in our group.

In order to achieve the best results, a more interdisciplinary approach to research concerning the fetus and newborn must be taken. A very good example is the problem of optimal drug dosages in premature and newborn babies. The only rational approach is to convince clinicians, pharmacologists, and other basic scientists to work together on the problem. However, in very few medical schools around the world has this interdisciplinary approach been followed. This is, perhaps, the reason why so little progress is currently accomplished in this field.

We build expensive intensive care units for premature and full-term newborn infants, but we really do not have the simple basic clinical knowledge of the optimal dosage of an antibiotic or digitalis to be given to these subjects, or the toxic effects that we could expect from various agents.

Finally, I would like to indicate that continuous collaboration between countries is most important. Collaboration can change in quality and form, but should, nonetheless, continue. The value of exchange between scientists of different backgrounds, different cultures, and different languages should be constantly fostered.

General Discussion

The discussion was opened by Behrman and Hellman who voiced confusion regarding the definition of the terms "perinatal and neonatal." It emanated from the discussion, particularly of Ransome-Kuti and Sir Dugald Baird, that differences existed between the British system and the American system by indicating that the word "perinatal" extended back to the 20th week when the Americans used the term and the 28th week when the British or Africans used the term. In evaluating "perinatal" or "neonatal" mortality, Ransome-Kuti cautioned against using hospital statistics. The basis for his admonition was that the hospital obstetric population is selective. He pointed out that what occurred in the home or in hospitals where the mothers were admitted for only 12 hours after delivery would result in an entirely different set of statistics.

Sereni asked Ransome-Kuti how, with the small neonatal units that exist in Nigeria, he, Ransome-Kuti, made the decision as to what babies should be admitted. Ransome-Kuti responded that the babies to be admitted were of course selected and the decision demanded considerable medical thought.

Longo voiced a plea for developing a system where doctors could fulfill military service time by helping in the developing countries. Ransome-Kuti responded by saying that this would be an excellent idea, but he, in his experience, was not in favor of forced service. He indicated that often there were many problems with forced service and that the people did not do as good a job as they might. He thought, however, that volunteer service would be a great help.

Ransome-Kuti brought up the problem of the necessity of education concerning breast-feeding in the developing countries, because there are social pressures placed on the women. More and more women are giving up breast-feeding earlier in the postnatal period. Greulich pointed out that the pressures of the social group are indeed important and cannot be ignored. Hellman asked whether there was sabotage to any of the educational programs inflicted by community or special groups. Ransome-Kuti said that it was necessary to develop rapport with the traditional doctor since he could sabotage the work in education. He hastened to add that the traditional doctor was very valuable in the treatment of psychiatric disorders.

O. J. Miller thought that statistics were important, but that it was imperative for the developing countries to recognize the numerous pitfalls. Consequently, he advised that the statistics should be gathered in a usable fashion and should be computerized.

Barnett spoke of the problem of communication between the developed and the developing world. He indicated that the best type of assistance is participation of a team from the developed world in the developing world where they could train people in technology. Ransome-Kuti said that he had such an association with groups at Stanford University and Johns Hopkins University and that it was working "very effectively." He went on to say that the roles were clearly defined. The Americans functioned to train his people, while he then was free to carry on the work while directing the work to those areas which were applicable and important to his country.

Gordon reiterated that there should be no competition between research and patient care. In fact, he stated, "I would like to see us stop talking about research versus care, because I think that research is the major determinant of the quality of what we are going to deliver for the cure of disease."

Sereni indicated that the world was dependent upon continuation of advanced and basic research by the affluent and semi-affluent nations. Those nations that did not have this affluence would, of course, have to borrow and parasitize the results and accumulated knowledge of affluent countries and utilize the information for care of patients. He underscored Gordon's comment and said that if research would dry up in the affluent nations, then this would have a precipitous effect on health care, not only locally but throughout the world. Rossi agreed emphatically with Sereni's statement. Discussion was initiated between Kretchmer and Hellegers concerning lack of communication between obstetricians and pediatricians. Hellegers made some comments on the extent of perinatologic work accomplished by obstetricians in Europe, particularly in Belgium and Holland. Kretchmer said that communication between obstetrics and pediatrics in the United States, as well as abroad, has been difficult and lacking. Barnett deplored the lack of importance that pediatrics has in the nations abroad and indicated that since obstetrics was a major specialty abroad, they might well take the prerogative in establishing lines of communication and mutual activity between the two specialties. Gordon indicated that there has been considerable progress over the past 15 years. Kretchmer stated that although the comment was true, progress had not been sufficient. Sereni indicated that not only is communication important but so are joint investigations. Metcalfe summarized the discussion and indicated that the pediatrician and obstetrician must learn to work together on problems involving perinatology. In fact, he pointed out that it is almost a question of survival for the two specialties, since the major problems in their fields are in the area of perinatal biology. Sir Dugald responded by saying that many of the problems that previously kept pediatricians busy are fast disappearing and they are now faced with the all-important problem of perinatology.

Gordon requested that Hasselmeyer discuss the problem of maternal-infant separation. Hasselmeyer responded by saying, "For a number of years, in my role as a nurse practitioner, I seriously questioned what nursery nurses did to newborn infants by the type of care rendered to them. For example, I was particularly concerned about the nursing practice of minimal handling and how this affected the baby's adaptation, growth, and development.

I have for many years been interested in the behavioral aspects of the newborn infant. I designed a study that challenged the nursing practice of minimal handling and evaluated the effects of sensory stimulation upon the general well-being of a group of prematurely-born infants. The theoretical foundation of the study was based upon Kulka's infancy kinesthetic need theory.

There were two groups of subjects, each consisting of 30 premature infants with birth weights between 1,501 and 2,000 g and who were between the ages of 7 and 13 days on admission to the sample. Each subject was studied for a 14-day period. One group of subjects received routine care and handling; the other group also received routine care but with amounts of handling and tactile and kinesthetic stimulation almost three times the amount received by the control group.

Analysis of the data revealed some interesting findings. One related to the weight gain of the babies. At the beginning of the study, infants in the high handling group weighed, on the average, less than the infants in the low handling-routine care group. By the end of two weeks, the weight curve of the group receiving increased amounts of handling had surpassed the low handling group. While the difference in the amount of weight gain was not statistically significant, there was a definite trend for more rapid weight gain in the high handling group.

I also found a difference in the frequency of minor infections. The group of babies that received the routine amount of handling had a greater incidence of minor infections than the group that received extra handling. Moreover, babies who received large amounts of handling and rocking were observed to be sleeping more, crying less, and they defecated less amount of feces. There may be a correlation here between the amount of sensory input received, enhanced oxygenation and metabolism, better utilization of food nutrients, and weight gain.

I also assessed frustration and stress levels of the babies at the beginning and end of their participation in the study. While there was no intergroup differences in these variables at the beginning of the study, I found that at the end of the two-week period, the babies receiving extrasensory input, as a group, showed less reactivity to frustration and stress tests than the babies cared for by the usual minimal handling routine.

This is just a brief resume. Some of this early work, perhaps, is responsible for challenging the present concepts of care of premature babies in the early weeks of life and studies concerned with its effect on later development.

Following this statement Gordon reiterated the importance of the nurse in the care of the infant. Minkowski underscored his statement and indicated that some studies were now in progress in Paris, and that in addition to the psychological problems of maternal-infant separation, there are also some nutritional and growth effects. The advantage of the freedom of the mother within the hospital, and her ability to join her infant in the hospital in the developing countries, was referred to by Gordon.

Hellman asked whether there was any evidence for an increase in the number of malformations in those areas which had been inundated with various pesticides. Minkowski responded by saying that certain pesticides such as 2,4,5-T and 2,4-D are associated with malformations in the rat. As a consequence, 2,4,5-T was withdrawn from the market. There is still no evidence in the human that there is an increase in malformations. Kretchmer suggested that there might be some possibility of statistical studies in the San Joaquin Valley where a great deal of various insecticides are utilized constantly. Kaiser indicated that there was a record of deaths resulting in agricultural workers from various insecticides, but to his knowledge there was no information concerning the pregnant woman. Since this is a very complicated field, involved with subjective reactions, James Miller advised caution and accumulation of hard data rather than emotional reactions.

The data on nutrition presented by Minkowski were questioned by Sereni who indicated that there was a possibility that some of the results could be explained by difference in ploidy in various cells. Ploidy would effect changes in DNA in the liver particularly but would have no effect on the brain. He said that the rat has been the major animal used for these studies and that the brain is not fully developed at birth in contrast to that of the mouse.

Dr. O. J. Miller indicated that if one really wanted to study neurological mechanisms, there was a great potentiality in utilizing organisms, other than vertebrates, for studies of basic mechanisms of neurological development. Kretchmer and James Miller pleaded for a broader use of the mouse for nutritional and developmental studies, since the genetics of the mouse was so well documented.

Summary and Implications

Summary and Implications

Louis M. Hellman

Summarizing a conference is indeed a difficult job. Those who have performed this task realize that one must give a learned and eloquent description of the proceedings. Furthermore, the group should be left with a sense of unity, with emphasis on the important points, in order to give a lasting impression of the conference.

The planners of this conference deserve praise. When Norman Kretchmer informed us about the agenda and the thoughts of the committee in selecting the various subjects, I wondered whether there would be any continuity.

Many of the participants were uneasy because, as scientists, data are usually presented in precise detail. This was not your task. Rather, you were asked to present your data briefly, only to make the major points, and not to prove your ability as a super investigator.

Some uneasiness did exist. I detected hesitancy to present complex slides. Dr. Minkowski probably best expressed his uneasiness when he had to superficially present very complicated data to make a point of importance. The experience was unique as well as valuable.

The conference did hold together. Some conclusions were drawn and these

I would like to discuss. Harry Gordon, in opening the conference, stressed several points. He stressed the need for better medical care and the dearth of research in perinatal biology. He pointed out the great dissatisfaction many of us have felt when our grants were approved but not funded.

He indicated the philosophies that separate us. It is to this point in particular that I wish to return in conclusion. Ted Quilligan, in the discussion, raised one more very important issue—the advantages and disadvantages of categorical grants.

Irwin Kaiser spoke for the minorities. All of us who work for the government are under orders to form committees to achieve racial, religious, age, and sexual balances. There are always people who question the results. The question of minority balance is perilous because it sometimes acts to the disadvantage of the segment of society it seeks to help. I would like to recommend a book that impressed me greatly. It is a newly published book: John Hersey's *A Letter to the Alumnae*. It is a must for those who are in academic in this time of unrest.

The conference considered environment and ecology. The two terms are really interchangeable; eco-system is somewhat more elaborate than environment. It has also highlighted perinatal research in Western Europe and Africa.

The motto of the conference, if one may be applied, can be attributed to Sir Dugald Baird when he said, "If you are going to have ten children, you have got to have what it takes." If that statement were universally applicable, everybody would be able to have ten children, if he or she were healthy. The effects on the population would be astonishing. Perhaps something would happen to our environment so that it would be undesirable to live at all.

In some respects, this conference has paid tribute to Sir Dugald Baird. He offered certain philosophies which brought to our attention unmeasurable social factors which play a vital role in the efficiency of human reproduction. His leadership in this field is attested to not only by what he has written, but by the group of people who chose to work with him—Raymond Ilsley, Angus Thompson, and Frank Hytten.

The significance of Sir Dugald Baird's work is that he has created a bridge between social science and pure science. The danger is that people can extract from and distort his conclusions for political benefit. Information derived from correlates has to be used in context in which it was formed. It is exceedingly dangerous, particularly in the political arena, if it is used to imply a cause and effect relationship.

Let us look at one example. President Kennedy used to say in an off-hand manner, "If I can get rid of poverty in the United States, two-thirds of all the mental retardation will disappear." The correlation is clear but the conclusion doubtful. Yet it certainly was beneficial for the housing industry, and it allowed him to spend public monies for a worthy cause. Perhaps that in itself is a good goal.

The sociological implications that Sanford Dornbusch presented were of interest. He discussed bridging the communication gap. He indicated that perhaps communication between patients and the givers of the health care was not as good as it should be. This conclusion appears valid.

Let us examine a correlation, but perhaps not a cause and effect situation. Of those nations that lead in low perinatal mortality, all have midwives who perform a large proportion of the deliveries. It has been my experience that, even with the best obstetricians or pediatricians, the communication between women and their physicians may be superficial compared to the communication that is established between one woman and another. One cannot conclude, however, that midwives reduce perinatal loss. Dr. Dornbusch talked about fashions of reproduction. The mores and ambitions of women change. This change has a profound effect on reproductive efficiency and on the health of the nation. The desire for small families in the United States is increasing. The ideal family is now under three. I would venture to say that in our pioneer days it was very close to five or seven.

He mentioned women's liberation. A lot of fun has been poked at this movement. I have been picketed by women, and it was indeed an uncomfortable experience. Nevertheless, I think that of the forces in operation in this country today, the women's liberation movement is going to be one of the most significant. The movement will alter women's views about the family, their role in the family, and other possible roles. If in fact we are going to control the rate of population growth in the United States, "women's liberation" is going to be extremely important, for it will furnish an alternative to marriage. This change is needed if the growth rate is to be diminished. Women's liberation will impel late marriage by substituting outside the home. All of these elements will have both positive and negative effects upon the way our society reproduces itself.

Dr. Dornbusch then discussed professors as a bureaucracy of professionals who are in but at the same time against the bureaucracy. I am reminded of Jerry Weisner's remark when he was the President's science advisor. He said, "The most valuable and most pleasant job in Washington is to be a consultant on leave from MIT." The problem has been that too few scientists have been willing to deal with the uncertainties and frustrations of the bureaucracy.

The result has been that the government has employed too few scientists. Two of the areas that attract nonscientists are health and science. Many of the decisions that vitally affect us are not made by scientific people but by a group of very bright young lawyers or people with other kinds of specialized training.

Dr. Dornbusch also mentioned professional evaluation. I would venture to say that we do a good job of evaluating research grants, with peer review, but when we try to evaluate medical care, we are up against an impossible situation. Expecting the medical professional to perform self-evaluation and to do something about its difficulties at the grass roots level is an unrealistic expectation.

The discussion of the sociological program was indeed interesting. Both multivariant and correlation approaches are extremely valuable and yield information that cannot be gathered in any other way. They are statistical techniques, however, and if they do not make things more simple and accurate, they are not useful in describing sociological phenomena.

Unfortunately, correlations in the field of reproduction very frequently are not accurate. Recently the collaborative study of cerebral palsy, upon which we have spent so much money, used the multivariant approach which resulted in misinformation.

I do not expect Alex Minkowski to be misled by statistical pitfalls, nor do I expect the professionals in this room to be misled. However, we must remember that the public can very easily be fooled by statistics, and sometimes investigators even deceive themselves. Unfortunately, it is easy to believe the information that comes from a very expensive computer.

I have written in my textbook that the purported relation between infection and prematurity, although extremely interesting, leaves the cause and effect relation unproved. I found Edward Kass extremely careful in qualifying his correlations. I believe Dr. Kass knows the limits to which his results can be pushed.

All of us would like a simplistic etiology for prematurity. It is extremely attractive that bacteria, their products, or viruses might be the sole etiologic agents. Dr. Kass' approach has a long history! Dr. Peters at Yale cited this theory over thirty years ago.

The discussion of rubella was of interest. The high altitude problem was introduced. We were presented with some clinical data, not well-controlled, but, in general, credible. If information does not make sense, one should review the sources. If it makes sense, it still must be controlled.

There are applicable techniques that have not been used in human research. For example, ultrasonographic techniques have been developed to ascertain the volume of the human placenta from about the fourteenth or fifteenth week of pregnancy to term. There are mathematical theories that relate volume to surface area. These techniques could be used, even in remote areas, to supplement the other kinds of data that were presented by Dr. Hellegers and by the group who did pioneer work in the Andes.

The relation of high altitude to hypoglycemia is of particular interest. It seems to me that high altitude research used a phenomenon of nature that will help us understand the homeostatic mechanisms that the placenta, the mother, and the baby use to combat stress. This is the crux of the situation. Our knowledge is still primitive. To give up high altitude research because so few people live at high altitudes, and because altitude does not affect very many people, is ridiculous.

Other types of stress were also discussed. Pollution is really a stressful situation that is with us all the time. The importance of the effect of pollution on reproductive efficiency is obvious. That the women in Nigeria breathe very high concentrations of carbon monoxide indoors is an interesting example. Maybe some of us in New York City are in equally bad condition. There are other areas of stress in our society. The chairman mentioned two—the heavy metals problem and the use of Merthiolate in an incubator which introduces a high concentration of mercury to the infant's air supply. We also have noise. Noise does affect the fetus, causing restlessness when loud noises or even bright lights are applied to the mother's abdomen.

What does crowding do to reproductive efficiency? Poverty and crowding usually go hand-in-hand, and we might answer this question if poverty could be separated from crowding. Population growth will produce crowding. It is important that we know some answers. There are a lot of theories about what crowding does to the political structure. People say, "Look what is happening in Calcutta. The government cannot function." Many of these conclusions are wishful thinking.

Finally, we approached genetics. Three priorities were mentioned. Dr. Rosenberg said that the three important things were differentiation, detection, and treatment. I think that we are on the verge of making intrauterine diagnoses at a rate and with an accuracy that were almost undreamed of ten years ago. These diagnoses will be not only genetic but they also will include abnormal metabolism. A host of conditions may be diagnosable before the decade is finished. If any choice were to be made concerning funding, this area should receive a heavy commitment.

As the population of the world begins to stabilize, and as smaller families emerge, there will be an increasing commitment that each child be as near-perfect as possible. This commitment is moral and absolute. One cannot say to the woman in India, "Don't have ten children," because she already knows some of them are going to die, but one might say to women in the United States, "Have only two children," because there is a reasonable chance that they will grow to maturity. If you could say, "We will also give you a reasonable assurance that the two you are going to have are going to be nearly perfect," we would have an inducement to limit family size.

Those were the conference highlights as I saw them.

Index

Prematurity, 52, 169
  and infection, 31, 32, 34, 48
Prematurity rates, 32
Primigravidae, 11, 13, 16, 18
Professional bureaucracy, 26
Proliferating cells, 135
Protoporphyrin, 63
Pyelonephritis, 35
  bacteria, 34
  chronic, 36
  pregnancy, 31
  symptomatic, 32

Quinacrine-fluorescence, 151
Quinacrine mustard and DNA, 151

Record linkage technology, 157
Regional differences in perinatal mortality
  rate, 14
Reproductive efficiency and environment,
  20
Research problems in genetics, 160
Respiratory disease, 56
Retinopathy, 34
Rh incompatibility, 168
Ribonucleic acid, see RNA
Richmond, Julius, 4
RNA, 124
  synthesis, 123, 135
Rubella, 42, 43, 45, 46, 48, 169
  and CNS, 47, 48
Rural health centers, 169

Sarrel study, 27
Screening, 125, 126
  for bacteriuria, 36
Sensory input, 179
Sickle cell trait, 123, 125
"Silent" congenital infections, 48, 49
Skeletal muscle and oxygen tension, 75
Small-for-dates animals, 172
Smoking, 80
Social barrier, 25
Socioeconomic groups, bacteriuria, 32, 39
  intrauterine infections, 45, 46
Socioeconomic levels, 13, 57, 85, 169
Spinal bifida, 81
Statistical evaluation, 173
Stillbirth rate, 19
  anencephaly, 16, 18
  ethnic factors, 19
Stillbirths, 167
Subependymal layer, 133, 134

Suburban health centers, 169
Sulfate pollutants, 56, 60
Sulfonamide and urine concentration, 35
Sulfur compounds, 57
Switzerland, 173
Symptomatic bacteriuria, 31
Symptomatic pyelonephritis, 32
Symptoms and practitioners, 24
Syphilis, 45, 46

Taboos, 167
Teens, pregnancy and social class, 27
Teratogenic factors, 127, 129, 135
Tetanus, 167, 168
Tetanus spores, 168
Tetracycline, 34, 36
  dental staining, 37
  in pregnant, bacteriuric patients, 34
  low birth weight, 37
Thermography, 72
Thymidine kinase locus, 152
Tissue culture, 160
Toxemia, 167
Toxoplasma and CNS, 47, 48
Toxoplasma infection, 42, 45, 49, 169
Toxoplasmosis, 46, 48
Translocation chromosomes, 151
Treponema Pallidum, 42
Trisomy and abortions, 152
Tritiated thymidine, 128, 131, 132, 135,
  136, 137, 139
Trypan blue, 129
Twinning, 167

United Kingdom, 15
Urinary concentration defect, 35
Urinary tract infections, 31
Urine culture, 36
Uterine artery, ligation of, 171

Vitamin A, 135

Wales, perinatal mortality, 16
Wilbur Report, 4
Witch doctors, 24
Women's liberation, 185

X chromosome, 124
X-irradiation, 135
X-irradiation and eye structure, 143

Yoruba, 167